## FROM THE EXPERTS

"Dr. Pagano has provided a new perspective in the management of psoriasis— one that justifies serious consideration by the scientific community."

*—Harold Mermelstein, MD,* dermatologist, New York, NY

"I am deeply impressed with your accomplishments in that dreaded condition called psoriasis. Where others have continued to fail, you have succeeded and your success is amazing and outstanding."

*—James F. Winterstein, DC,* president,
the National University of Health Sciences, Lombard, IL

"Dr. Pagano's book *Healing Psoriasis: The Natural Alternative* firmly convinces me that he has achieved a phenomenal success in the healing arts—a humane accomplishment. I think it merits world attention. How many poor souls must be waiting in the wings for such a blessed, humanitarian gift!"

*—Peter Henderson, EdD*, author/journalist/educator, Haworth, NJ

"John Pagano's book is nothing less than spectacular. Psoriasis, eczema, acne, and practically all skin conditions are reflections of inner metabolic imbalances, which, in turn, are the result of numerous diet, toxin, and lifestyle stresses. The conventional medical approach is to suppress the immune system by immunosuppressive drugs and corticosteroids. The good news is that there is a safe, effective, and very scientific way of reversing these skin problems naturally. The Pagano treatment goes to the root of the problem, provides natural anti-inflammatory relief, and prevents recurrences. The medical literature supports the use of many aspects of Pagano's approach. The proof of its efficacy is plain to see in the thousands of individuals rescued from a life of misery. This book is must reading for all dermatologists, family doctors, naturopaths, and their patients with chronic skin disorders."

*—Zoltan P. Rona, MD, MSc,* medical editor,
*The Encyclopedia of Natural Healing*, Toronto, Ontario, Canada

"I have viewed the evidence; I have met Dr. Pagano's patients—it works! This book should encourage further research not only in psoriasis and the dermatoses, but in other devastating illnesses. Responsible researchers would do well to seriously investigate this material for what it has to offer suffering humanity."

*—Faina Munits, MD, PhD,* West Orange, NJ

"Dr. Pagano is a gift of God to millions who suffer from the terrible disease of psoriasis, which allopathic doctors all over the world regard as incurable. Dr. Pagano has proven that, through a change of diet and by following a strict regimen, psoriasis can be cured.

His book, *Healing Psoriasis: The Natural Alternative,* deserves to be translated into different languages and published in many countries. It is so packed with healthy information that it will be read with profit, not merely by those afflicted with psoriasis, but by all who aspire to live a happy, healthy, harmonious life.

—*Dada J. P. Vaswani,* head of Sadhu Vaswani Mission, Pune, India

## FROM THE PATIENTS

*Mrs. R.M.T. of Lindenwold, NJ:* "We heard about your success treating psoriasis. At the first visit, you explained the disease. I left your office with a new, positive attitude and a great outlook on life. In three months we could see a remarkable improvement. At nine months, I was clear of lesions. Now I am walking on air, because we have the psoriasis under control. It was you and the wonderful book you have written. I'm glad I chose the alternative path."

*Mrs. J.H. of South Australia:* "I have suffered from pustular psoriasis for over twenty-two years, and not once did the skin specialist I was going to *ever* mention that what I may be eating could be a cause. I tried everything, from pills and creams, natural methods such as being wrapped in comfrey leaves, PUVA treatments, and so on. I came across your book and I couldn't believe it. Here was a book that made sense. I can now say that some areas have cleared up completely and my left palm (which is the last patch) is clearing up. Many, many, many thanks. I am so happy with what I have managed to do *myself.*"

*Mr. J.W. of Salem, OR:* "Who do you believe? A scientist who has never been plagued with psoriasis every day of his miserable life for X amount of years, or someone who has? You deserve the Nobel Peace Prize for helping so many good people. Those children in your book are the most touching of all, especially young L. Again, Dr. Pagano, thank you very much."

# Healing
# Psoriasis

# Healing
# Psoriasis

## THE NATURAL ALTERNATIVE

John O. A. Pagano, DC

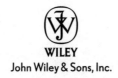

**WILEY**
John Wiley & Sons, Inc.

To my beautiful sisters,
Carol and Maria,
and
to the memory of
my devoted parents,
Nettie Pagano and John J. Pagano, Esq.,
and
my white German Shepherd,
Shane

# CONTENTS

Foreword by Harry K. Panjwani, MD, PhD      xi
Preface      xiii

1. Psoriasis: The "Inside" Story      1
2. Does the Regimen Work?      11
3. About Psoriasis      17
4. The Natural Alternative      32
5. Internal Cleansing      36
6. Diet and Nutrition Basics      67
7. Herbal Teas      111
8. The Role of the Spine      119
9. External Applications      129
10. Right Thinking: The Role of the Mind      145
11. The Emotional Factor      160
12. The Crowning Glory      172
13. Psoriasis on the Hands, the Feet, and the Nails      180
14. The Healing Process      194
*A Photographic Portfolio*      201
15. Pushing the Panic Button      215
16. The Arthritic Connection: Psoriatic Arthritis      222

17. Cases of Eczema (Atopic Dermatitis) 238

18. What about the Failures? 250

19. The Question of Recurrence 257

20. Achieving the Goal: A Mini-Review 262

21. Where Do We Go from Here? 267

Appendix A.  Nutritional Considerations in
the Natural Healing of Psoriasis, Eczema,
and Psoriatic Arthritis 272

Appendix B.  Menu Plans and Recipes 283

Appendix C.  Self-Hypnosis Recording for the Psoriatic 303

Appendix D.  Product Suppliers 306

Acknowledgments 307

Notes 308

Bibliography 312

Illustration Credits 315

Index 317

# FOREWORD

by Harry K. Panjwani, MD, PhD

The concept of this rather unique and unusual book is to emphasize the power of the human organism to heal the body, with the help of proper diet, posture, and gait; attitude; and internal cleansing, thus removing the toxins that cause diseases. The regimen outlined in this book pertains to psoriasis—a devastating, humiliating skin disease, usually chronic and recurrent in nature, that often leads to depression, despair, and other health problems as well as isolation, and certainly to interference with the sufferer's personal and family life, as well as employment and enjoyment of life in general.

There are many references to dietary restrictions for health in the Old Testament. The use of herbs in food or drink is a common practice in Eastern countries like India, China, and Japan. For centuries, internal cleansing, fasting, and other methods have been a common practice in European spas to remove toxins from the body. External cleansing is also important, considering the elements to which our skin is exposed throughout the day, in addition to the psychological and cosmetic importance of clean skin.

We, of course, must pay attention to habits and lifestyle, sleep patterns, our environment, and our emotions. The biomechanics of the body—posture and gait—are very important. We have learned in recent years that alternate approaches to health care are being successfully utilized in treating cancer, diabetes, coronary artery disease, stroke, arthritis, depression, and other diseases.

It is essential to ascertain the safety of any treatment and not to overlook other known methods of treatment. This certainly applies to the treatment of psoriasis outlined in this book. In addition to the physical and emotional requirements, we need the open-mindedness, the personal sense of morality, and the spiritual outlook to round off the total approach.

Biofeedback has been in use for many years. It confirms that we can effect biochemical changes in our body when necessary. We need to assume responsibility for our individual health while also recognizing our capacity for self-healing.

I wholeheartedly recommend this book to the psoriatic or his family, to health professionals, and to other interested parties for the information it offers.

# PREFACE

## A New Beginning

When a thing is understood, the cure is half accomplished.
— Anne Shannon Monroe

On June 10, 1997, one week before I began my European speaking tour, the following e-mail came to my office from a Mr. Charles Shannon of St. Albans, West Virginia:

> I am sixty-eight years of age, and for sixty-three years of my life, I have suffered with psoriasis. Every method has been tried, from tar baths to PUVA [psoralen-ultraviolet light A], being in the trial government study of the PUVA method. The disease always came back more severely—sometimes covering 80 percent of my body. I ordered the book [*Healing Psoriasis: The Natural Alternative*] on February 27, 1997. After receiving the book, I started reading and getting the supplies ready. I really started the diet toward the end of March 1997. Now, three months later, I can't believe the results. My skin is almost completely healed! I have followed the regimen— diet, etc.; I even stopped smoking. When I started, my back looked like the *before* picture on the back cover of your book. My legs healed first, then my back, stomach, face—the arms were the last. I would like to thank you wholeheartedly. No scales—no itching— no bleeding. I feel as if I can wear a short-sleeve shirt with peace of mind, for the first time in my life. May God bless you and thank you so much for caring!

Mr. Shannon followed the suggestions in the first edition of my book and was practically 100 percent clear of psoriasis in less than three months, after having suffered with it for sixty-three years! However, let's be realistic. This is an unusually successful case, considering the many years he had the disease and how quickly he cleared up.

Unsolicited letters, e-mails, and reports like this one have come into my office from every part of the globe since my book was first published in 1991. The reason for such results is that I use an approach to the disease that the scientific community has never taken before. The path I have followed for forty years is one that views the problem of psoriasis from the inside out rather than the outside in. The answer to the riddle of psoriasis will never be found by focusing the attention on the skin. We must go inside to seek origins and look for causes that once found and understood put the patients on the road to recovery, provided they are willing to cooperate.

The purpose of this volume is to bring a ray of hope to the tens of millions of people worldwide who suffer from psoriasis, one of mankind's oldest, most elusive, chronic inflammatory skin diseases. This hope is not based merely on theory and speculation, but on solid, concrete evidence of results obtained by following a regimen of therapy I have developed over the major part of my professional career.

During this time, particularly in the past thirty years, I have concentrated my efforts on proving, indisputably, that psoriasis—long classified as "incurable" by the scientific community—can be healed in a perfectly natural way. The method I have developed is devoid of any systemic or topical drug (they often have harmful side effects), uncomfortable messy tar baths, or even potentially dangerous forms of ultraviolet light. In short, I contend that psoriasis is one incurable disease that the patient does not necessarily have to live with. In many cases it is possible for every psoriatic lesion, rash, or abrasion to completely disappear, leaving the patient in control of the problem throughout his or her entire life. That is the message of this book and the purpose for which it was written.

It may come as a surprise to many that I, a chiropractic physician, have taken it upon myself to investigate this dermatological enigma that for centuries has frustrated researchers who were seeking a cause and a cure. It may come as even more of a surprise to learn that the results I have obtained were achieved by practicing well-known, time-honored principles and techniques that fall completely under the heading of natural or holistic healing. In other words, I am utilizing natural methods, in a new way, on an old disease.

It is not my intention in any way to minimize the efforts of dedicated researchers and physicians in the field of dermatology. Clearly, they have made life more bearable for many victims of the disease through endless research and various therapies they have developed. Rather, it is my desire to share with them the results I have obtained, by revealing the methods I used when attacking this disease from a different perspective—from the inside out, as opposed to from the outside in.

Since the cause and true cure for psoriasis remain unknown in the field of dermatology, I ask merely that these findings be taken into consideration. Without question, further research is needed under better controlled conditions; but, given the facts contained here, perhaps a new beginning emerges in understanding the disease that will justify such research. I submit that the information presented here warrants such investigation.

The approach to psoriasis that I have used is based on the works of Edgar Cayce (1877–1945), a remarkable individual whose discourses on healing are legendary and are becoming more popular with each passing year. Using his advanced theory as a guide to understanding the cause of the disease, as well as a suggested regimen of therapy, I have combined my clinical experience and slowly evolved a working hypothesis, a natural alternative that, over the years, has proven to be extremely beneficial in many cases. I have shown that when psoriasis is understood from this new perspective, faith in the process is strengthened by logic and reason—or, to put it more succinctly, "It makes sense!" as so many patients have said.

Unquestionably there have been failures, as there are in all research projects. In practically every case, however, the reason for failure was found to be the patient's own impatience. Outstanding results were not achieved overnight. Most patients who succeeded in ridding themselves of psoriasis did so by giving a great deal of time and honest effort and, above all, being persistent. Without these invaluable mental ingredients, healing is not only difficult, it is impossible. Unless a patient is *committed* to freeing himself of this disfiguring disease, the efforts of both the patient and the physician are ultimately futile.

It does not necessarily follow, however, that success is guaranteed; but with dedication to the regimen, the chances are infinitely greater. To this day, when success is achieved, I am amazed to see how a patient's skin can renew itself totally and completely, without even a trace of the devastating lesions that once covered the body. I believe it *can* be done for the simple reason that it *has* been done. This is not speculation; it is a declaration, the proof of which is found in the pages that follow.

The late Gina Cerminara, PhD, author and lecturer, once told me, quite aptly, that "the secret of good writing is to be understood." For this reason, I have endeavored to keep it simple, so my readers may grasp the underlying principles of the nature of the disease. Consequently, sophisticated medical terminology was purposely kept to a minimum. I hope I have succeeded.

Within the pages of this book, psoriasis may be understood for what it is, and with this understanding comes the hope that despite present conditions, a natural healing is possible. It is my ardent wish that this is so, for then psoriasis sufferers can begin putting their lives in order and get on with the business of living, no longer burdened under the yoke of this disfiguring, all-consuming disease.

This book was first released in May 1991 at the Edgar Cayce Center in Virginia Beach, Virginia. The very first bookstore to carry it was the little Monmouth Beach Book Shop on the Jersey Shore, where I was raised. Now, years later, orders for the book come in from virtually every country on Earth. Psoriasis is a global affliction with more than a hundred million people wrapped in its clutches. If ten people can be helped by taking the approach outlined in this book, then a hundred can; if a hundred, then a thousand; if a thousand, then why not millions? With only a minimum of advertising, the book grows in popularity simply by word of mouth, the most effective way to determine the value of a book. I sincerely thank the many sufferers who have read the book and spread the word. I also thank those who have taken the time to write or contact me to express their overwhelming gratitude. There is no greater reward for this physician turned author than the results of his labors manifested in such a glorious way.

At the time of this writing, *Healing Psoriasis: The Natural Alternative* is in its seventh printing and has sold over fifty thousand copies in the

United States and around the world. It has been the number-one best seller in its category with both Amazon.com and BarnesandNoble.com for the past nine consecutive years. To date, it has been translated into Russian, Italian, Finnish, and Japanese. This is a far cry from humble beginnings in the early 1970s, when my first case of psoriasis walked into my office and was healed in a matter of a few months, changing the course of the patient's life and mine.

Now, John Wiley & Sons, of Hoboken, New Jersey, has taken over publishing rights to the book. With this honor granted me, the third phase of one of Edgar Cayce's directives is about to be fulfilled. "First," he said, "go to the individual, then to the groups, and then to the masses." With John Wiley & Sons, the book can now reach the millions of psoriasis victims with a message of hope for the healing of a disease that has plagued mankind probably since the dawn of history.

This eighth year of the new millennium marks my forty-eighth year in active clinical practice as a chiropractic physician. It has been a rewarding adventure—the joy of healing patients goes far beyond what words can express. But it is time to move on to new adventures; not to retire, but to aspire. There is much more for me to do before I check out here and check in there!

It has given me indescribable joy and an enormous sense of accomplishment to have played a part in this revelation. I have always been of the opinion that mankind was not put on this earth to suffer but to live. The misery that plagues man is of his own making, through ignorance, selfishness, greed, and an unprecedented disregard for natural laws. Know the natural laws and respect and adhere to them, and sickness and disease will vanish. *This is our natural heritage.* Psoriasis is only one of the diseases mankind is burdened with, but with the evidence presented here, as far as psoriasis and eczema are concerned, I would say we are off to a pretty good start.

# CHAPTER 1

# Psoriasis: The "Inside" Story

Doctor, you must help me—I can no longer go on living this way." These were the first words Mr. A. uttered to me as I greeted him at my door. He was a friendly, pleasant man in his late sixties. Judging by his outward appearance, one would assume there wasn't a thing wrong with him. But something was indeed wrong—radically wrong. When Mr. A. disrobed, I saw the reason for his torment. He was a victim of one of mankind's oldest skin diseases: psoriasis. He had been suffering with the disease for thirty years. It had finally reached a point where over 80 percent of his body was covered with thickened, silvery scales that caused pain, bleeding, and intolerable itching.

He had heard about me from a local health food store owner, who told him that I had helped several psoriasis sufferers. Mr. A, having exhausted all other available means of fighting the disease, came to me with the expectation that I might solve his problem.

His case was so severe that I hesitated to accept him as a patient, for fear of giving him false hope. I had no choice, however, when he pleaded, "Doctor, I have no one else to turn to."

I am happy that he persuaded me to accept him as a patient, for he proved to be totally cooperative. He followed my instructions to the letter, and much to my (and his) surprise, he was totally clear of all lesions in thirty days!

This patient was, and still is, the fastest-responding case I have ever witnessed. Most patients take from three to six months to show results. Years later, Mr. A appeared before a group of my patients to verify his successful recovery. He was an inspiration to all who met him.

Mr. A's success had come about by following a regimen of therapy based on a theory never before recognized or even seriously considered by the scientific community. This theory accounts for his success and the success of many others whom I have had the privilege of treating.

## My Definition of Psoriasis

Since psoriasis has often been described but never really defined, I offer this as a reasonable definition of the disease, based on my many years of clinically dealing with the subject: *Psoriasis is the external manifestation of the body's attempt to "throw off" internal toxins.* In other words, to put it more succinctly, the skin is doing what the bowels and the kidneys *should* be doing. The skin is not ordinarily designed to remove waste matter to any great extent, but, due to the toxic overload produced by a leaky gut, it acts as a backup system and takes on the task of removing toxins—thus the rash, irritation, and lesions.

## The Cause of Psoriasis

Looking to the skin for the cause of psoriasis is like looking at the tip of an iceberg and assuming it to be the entire structure. One can keep chipping away at the tip, but the iceberg will never disappear. Why? Because its main body lies hidden beneath the surface, and as long as that remains hidden, the iceberg will continue to exist.

So it is with psoriasis. What one sees on the outside is the physical evidence of something happening *inside* the body. One can treat the outside, but the disease will keep coming back again and again, month after month, year after year, until the patient has exhausted all available avenues of relief. Whom does he turn to? Is there really a remedy to this irritating, often devastating, chronic skin disease? Is it possible for a victim to be free from a lifetime of pain, disfigurement, and considerable expense?

The answer to these questions is an unequivocal yes! There are solutions to the riddle of psoriasis, solutions that have guided me in effectively managing the disease in a safe, natural way.

If a researcher turns to orthodox medicine for an explanation of the cause of this disease, he will still be met today with the same age-old declaration that "there is no known cause or cure for psoriasis." Only an inner belief that there *must* be an answer, although presently unknown, will motivate this scientist to continually seek a solution.

I have done just that by turning to the works of Edgar Cayce, where I found what sounded like a logical explanation for the disease. "There is a cure," declared Cayce. He then went on to cite the cause and suggest a remedy. The question remained, however, could his theories be proven? This led me into concentrated research for a period of fifteen years. During that time, I convinced my patients, as well as myself, that the information provided by Cayce was indeed valid and worthy of serious consideration in the treatment and management of the disease. In this book, Cayce's information and the concepts drawn from it are revealed as clearly and as simply as possible. Simple, however, does not necessarily mean easy. It all depends on the attitude of the patient. What is easy for one person may seem monumentally difficult to another. I advise my patients to approach the problem in a relaxed, confident way. Anxiety is not part of the regimen.

As an example of the effect of attitude, the skin of one of my patients cleared up in fourteen months after his suffering with psoriasis for fourteen years. He expressed his gratitude when he said, "Fourteen months after fourteen years is not bad." Eight years after his skin cleared, he remained satisfied with his results.

Another patient, after staying on the regimen for two weeks, complained, "Had I known it was this difficult, I would have never started." Needless to say, she remains a victim of psoriasis.

In order for the treatment to work the patient must first understand psoriasis for what it is; second, it is important to get on the right track, to rid oneself of the disease; and third, the patient must have patience and persistence!

## The Origin of Psoriasis

As mentioned earlier, to understand the reason for the outward manifestations of psoriasis, one must go inside the body to find the origin. According to the theories advanced by Cayce, that source is found in the *intestinal tract.* Here is where psoriasis begins and, until this fact is fully grasped and therapy is based on this premise, I believe with utmost certainty that the condition will persist.

For psoriasis to occur, the walls in certain areas of the intestinal tract must become thin and porous. When this happens, toxic substances that should normally pass through the intestines and eventually be eliminated by the body seep through these walls, enter the lymphatic system, and invade the bloodstream. The body's natural purification system, primarily the liver and the kidneys, then tries to filter out these toxins, which build up in the blood. It may take some time, but sooner or later the accumulation of toxins will prove to be more than these organs can effectively handle. When this point is reached, the body's secondary or backup purification systems attempt to aid in the process of elimination. When the liver, the major filtering gland of the body, is overloaded, the skin comes to the rescue and helps to eliminate toxins. When the kidneys are overtaxed, the lungs come into play. This concept is clearly explained in the works of Henry Bieler, MD, and is discussed in a later chapter.

## A Brief Anatomy Lesson

The digestive tract, the area primarily involved in the origin of psoriasis, is actually a long tube that carries out various functions all along its course, from the ingestion of food to the elimination of waste products.

When food enters the mouth, certain enzymes begin the process of breaking it down for eventual absorption and assimilation in the small intestine. Before food reaches the twisting and turning small intestine, it must pass down a straight section of tubing called the *esophagus* and enter the stomach. There it may remain for hours, being acted upon by more enzymes and certain acids before passing into the first portion of the small intestine, the *duodenum,* which is only about twelve inches long.

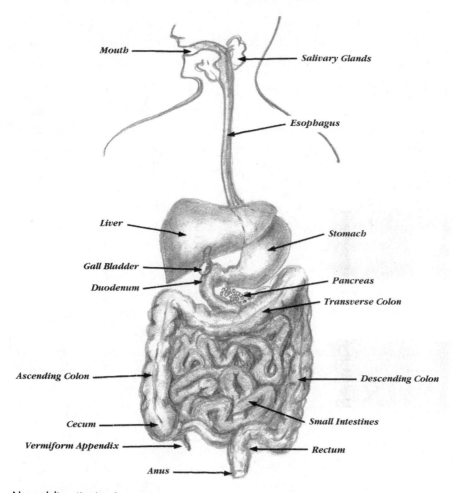

Mouth

Salivary Glands

Esophagus

Liver

Stomach

Gall Bladder

Duodenum

Pancreas

Transverse Colon

Ascending Colon

Descending Colon

Cecum

Small Intestines

Vermiform Appendix

Rectum

Anus

Normal digestive tract.

It then enters the next portion of the small intestine, called the *jejunum*, which, in turn, leads into the *ileum*.

It is within these areas, especially where the duodenum meets the jejunum, that the walls of the intestines in the psoriatic become thin and smooth, allowing a transfer of toxins to take place. This transferance can, however, take place anywhere along the entire length of the alimentary canal. This is called *intestinal permeability,* commonly referred to as the leaky gut syndrome.

## The Leaky Gut Syndrome Explained

To facilitate understanding of the leaky gut syndrome, I refer to the impressive work of Zoltan P. Rona, MD, MSC, of Toronto, Canada, who gives the following concise description of this now recognized disease:

> The Leaky Gut Syndrome is the name given to a very common health disorder in which the basic organic defect (lesion) is an intestinal lining which is more permeable (porous) than normal. The abnormally large spaces present between the cells of the gut wall allow the entry of toxic material into the bloodstream that would, in healthier circumstances, be repelled and eliminated. The gut becomes leaky in the sense that bacteria, fungi, parasites and their toxins, undigested protein, fat and waste, normally not absorbed into the bloodstream in the healthy state, pass through a damaged, hyperpermeable, porous, or leaky gut.

Dr. Rona states that the leaky gut syndrome "is almost always associated with autoimmune disease, and reversing autoimmune disease depends on healing the lining of the gastrointestinal tract." He named diseases in this category, such as lupus, rheumatoid arthritis, multiple sclerosis, fibromyalgia, chronic fatigue syndrome, vertigo, Crohn's disease, ulcerative colitis, and diabetes, among others, as being directly related to a hyperpermeable intestinal wall. With leaky gut problems, we become less resistant to viruses, bacteria, parasites, and candida (yeast infections). These are but a few of the many diseases or conditions that are now being closely scrutinized as having their origin in a leaky gut.

I find it interesting that Edgar Cayce was the first to offer this explanation for the cause of psoriasis, over sixty years ago. He described this osmotic process, which takes place in the intestines, as seepage of toxins through thin intestinal walls. Although he did not refer to it specifically as "intestinal permeability" or "leaky gut," it is quite obvious that he was describing the same phenomenon using the language of his day.

## Why the Walls Break Down

Dr. Rona lists the following causes associated with the breakdown of the intestinal walls that produces the leaky gut syndrome:

- *Antibiotics,* because they lead to the overgrowth of abnormal flora in the gastrointestinal tract (bacteria, parasites, candida, fungi)

- *Alcohol and caffeine,* which are strong gut irritants
- *Foods and beverages contaminated by parasites*
- *Chemicals* in fermented and processed foods
- *Enzyme deficiencies*
- *Prescription corticosteroids* (Prednisone)
- A *diet high in refined carbohydrates* (for example, candy bars, cookies, cake, soft drinks, white bread)
- *Prescription hormones* (birth-control pills)
- *Mold and fungal mycotoxins* in stored grains, fruit, and refined carbohydrates

I would also add the following, each of which will be dealt with as we proceed:

- *Chronic constipation*
- *Improper elimination*
- *Insufficient daily intake of water*
- *Foods high in saturated fat*
- *The "nightshades,"* particularly tomatoes, which carry an enzyme that is powerfully destructive to the psoriatic, eczematous, and arthritic patient
- *Smoking*
- *Negative emotions* such as resentment, fear, and anxiety
- *Depression*
- *Spinal misalignments*
- *Hereditary factors*

## Rebuilding the Walls

As you can see, there are many reasons that the intestinal walls break down and become porous. The good news is that the repair and regeneration of these walls is well within the reach of the average person, for the inner *lumen* (wall) that forms the barrier that prevents undesirable elements from seeping through is normally renewed and regenerated every six days—provided, of course, that consumption of irritants is halted and other beneficial substances are introduced.

The two primary substances taken internally, which I have used successfully, are *slippery elm bark powder* and *American yellow saffron tea.*

Both are prepared in the form of a tea and are administered with the purpose of healing the internal walls of the intestine and purifying the entire alimentary canal. (These teas may be obtained by calling Baar Products at 1-800-269-2502, online at www.baar.com, or contacting the Heritage Store at 1-800-862-2923, online at www.heritage@caycecures.com.)

## The Folds throughout the Intestinal Tract

The food, known as *chyme* at this stage of digestion, continues to move into the ileum, the longest portion of the approximately twenty-three-foot-long small intestine, where nutrients are absorbed and waste matter is passed into the large intestine and then the colon and is eventually eliminated.

The walls throughout most of the intestinal tract should have certain folds present at all times, aiding in the absorption and movement of

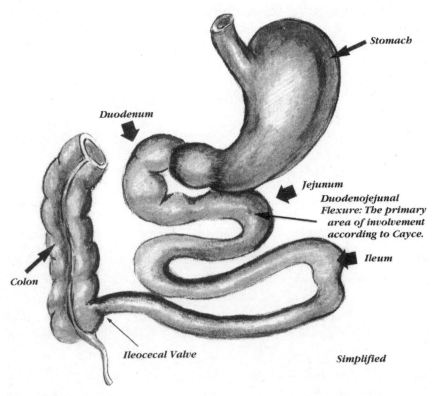

The starting point.

the contents that are passing through. These folds begin at the latter half of the duodenum, continue throughout the jejunum, and end about halfway into the ileum. They are more concentrated at the duodenojejunal flexure.

According to the information supplied by Cayce, when these folds become smooth, as though they were thinned out in the psoriatic, they permit a seepage of toxins through the walls and eventually into the bloodstream. Anatomically, they are called the *plicae circulares* (valves of Kerckring).

Although the transfer of toxins occurs primarily at the duodenojejunal flexure, this seepage of poisons can and probably does take place throughout the length of both the small and large intestines of a person suffering from psoriasis. The idea, therefore, in this new approach to the disease is twofold: (1) to cut down or preferably stop ingesting pollutants, and (2) to strengthen these porous intestinal walls.

## Why the Intestinal Walls Become Thin

In his 1968 treatise for the Medical Research Division of the Edgar Cayce Foundation, Frederick D. Lansford Jr., MD, reported that the smoothing of the intestinal walls does not always have the same cause, but more often than not is due to improper coordination in the eliminating systems.

Doubtless, some of the conditions that cause poor elimination overlap each other, contributing to a toxic buildup and causing an increase in acids in the blood that should always be alkaline. The acid content of the blood must be reduced. This is the basis for the therapeutic regimen outlined in the subsequent chapters of this book.

The toxic buildup I refer to is caused by not only those elements that have already been identified as having a poisonous effect on the body, such as carbon monoxide, nitrogen oxides, hydrocarbons, cyclamates, and many others, but there are also other substances that are more common but less suspect, especially certain foods that do not necessarily affect the average person but play havoc with the psoriatic. They act as allergens to psoriasis suffers and turn their lives into a living hell. The control of the disease, therefore, is attained primarily by learning to identify those foods that cause a toxic overacidic reaction in the body and by making it a priority to avoid them at all costs.

## Why the Intestinal Walls Become Porous

When the intestinal walls are already thin and compromised, they are more susceptible to fungal yeast infections. Yeast that collects in the folds of the intestinal villi (due to overly acidic pH levels that result from eating too many yeast-laden foods, especially sugar and white flour products, or from overuse of antibiotics) can change from normal, beneficial yeast into fungal yeast. This new fungal yeast grows roots (rhizoids) that penetrate the gut wall in their search for nutrition derived from blood, thus opening passageways for the toxic macromolecules to invade the blood circulatory system. The resulting "pinholes" are the source of the term "leaky gut." The waste matter or toxins that should ordinarily pass out of the body can now find a passageway into the blood. Remove the fungal yeast buildup and the gut will heal, preventing further leakage into the blood. This is best done by avoiding the foods that basically caused the problem—too many carbohydrates and sugars—and instead consume foods that help correct the problem—olive oil and garlic, as well as plain, organic yogurt with live cultures—and the chances of recovery are greatly enhanced. For information on testing for intestinal permeability (leaky gut), have your physician contact Genova Diagnostics at 1–800–522–4762.

# Understanding the Connection

Until this concept of nutritional effects on the skin is fully understood, one fights a losing battle. External applications in the form of salves, creams, and even ultraviolet light do help in many cases to clear the skin, but they are palliative at best, and before long, the condition usually returns, often worse than before. To those relatively few who have experienced a spontaneous remission of the disease without ever having a return of symptoms, I say they should thank their lucky stars. For reasons that may never be known, these fortunate few were relieved of a lifetime of anxiety and pain.

To those less fortunate, however, I say, take heart! All is not lost. There is a way out of your dilemma—a natural one that has been proven to be successful in many cases. It is a joy to my patients, as well as to me, to share the knowledge of this alternative path with you in the pages that follow.

# CHAPTER 2

# Does the Regimen Work?

My interest in psoriasis actually began while I was an intern in Denver, Colorado. The first case I saw, Mr. D.H., was a pleasant, enthusiastic dairy farmer from southern New Jersey. Since we were from the same state, a friendship as well as a doctor-patient relationship evolved. Although little could be done for his condition at that time, he came every year to the hospital in Denver to take advantage of the bright, sunlit days of Colorado. He said it always helped to clear his skin, if only temporarily. His twenty-year battle with psoriasis touched me so deeply that I took a keen interest in learning all I could about the disease. Little did I realize that fifteen years would pass before I would meet Mr. D.H. again at his home in New Jersey, where I would show him the successful results I had attained on my early cases.

In the interim, I kept gathering any information I could on psoriasis. Nothing seemed to hold much promise until I investigated the files on the disease available to me as a member of the Edgar Cayce Foundation in Virginia Beach, Virginia. (The Edgar Cayce Foundation is the sister organization of the Association for Research and Enlightenment [ARE], headquarters for the Cayce material.) The numerous files are made available to serious researchers, the over thirty-one thousand members, as well as the general public.)

I carefully studied the two volumes on psoriasis in the circulating files and proceeded to condense the information into a practical working order. "Why not?" I thought. Since orthodox medicine was still groping for answers, the question remained open. As so aptly stated by Norman Cousins, the author of the national best seller *Anatomy of an Illness,* "The art of healing is still a frontier profession." I proceeded to break down the information and convert it into a practical application. No sooner had I formulated a working hypothesis than my first psoriasis case walked in.

Actually, Mr. William Culmone came to me because of a spinal problem, not psoriasis. (Note that special permission has been granted to use Mr. Culmone's full name.) When he disrobed for his initial examination, my reaction was disbelief. Here was an unmistakable, rather severe case of psoriasis. I decided I would only record the fact that he had psoriasis, rather than discuss it with a new patient at our first meeting. My efforts were concentrated on his spinal problem, which gradually subsided and then disappeared. During each visit, as we spoke, I touched upon my studies in psoriasis and my source of information and slowly aroused his interest. By the time his back problem cleared up, he was ready to join me in an experiment, using this new approach to healing psoriasis.

Mr. Culmone had tried just about everything for over fifteen years, without results. His was a typical case of common psoriasis with bleeding, itching, scaling, and all else that accompanies this form of the disease. On July 21, 1975, we began the regimen with the full cooperation of his wife, Minnie. With specific instructions in his possession, he left the office and was told to return in one week.

He came back at the appointed time, disrobed in the examining room, and showed me his lesions. I was astonished at the results; they were at least 50 percent improved. Obviously, healing was taking place. The large lesion on his right thigh and several on the lumbar area of his spine were now a light pink color, with no scales. They were a far cry from the bloody, crusty patches of seven days earlier.

It took about three months, but on October 16, 1975, Mr. Culmone was no longer a victim of psoriasis. All lesions had disappeared as completely as if someone had used an eraser on his back.

He agreed to put the records of his case on display at the Edgar Cayce Foundation Library, in the hope that psoriasis sufferers who saw them would consider following the regimen, which I had worked out from the information supplied in the Cayce material. Exhibited with his case history and photographs in a special glass-enclosed display at the library (along with those of several other patients of mine), is Mr. Culmone's signed affidavit, which reads:

To Whom It May Concern:

RE: Psoriasis Report

This is to verify that the photographs presented in this report, as well as the sequence in which they were taken, were, in fact, taken at the specified intervals reported herein at the office of Dr. John O. A. Pagano.

The psoriasis I have suffered with for the past fifteen years has virtually "cleared up" in a period of three months, from the start of treatment. I can honestly state that there has been no recurrence whatsoever.

William Culmone

Mr. Culmone remained clear of all lesions for the remainder of his life. He died of unrelated causes. He will always remain in my memory as the first patient who was healed of psoriasis by following this new, natural approach to healing the disease. Mr. Culmone contributed much to all psoriasis victims by his unselfish attitude and willingness to discipline himself.

Patient:    William Culmone
Age:        65 years
Afflicted:  15 years

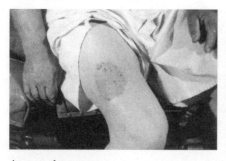 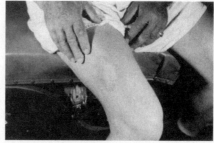

At start of regimen.                 Less than 3 months later.

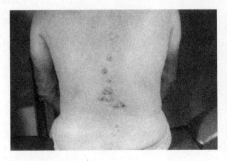
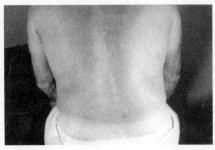

At start of regimen.                            Less than 3 months later.

## The Early Cases

My next severe case was that of Mrs. B.K., whose condition took four months to clear up. Then came the case of a little boy, A.S., who also responded beautifully in four months. After that was E.L., a little girl, who took about three months. Others followed in rapid succession. The die was cast; my destiny was set. I knew I had to continue with my research until it culminated in incontrovertible evidence that this approach did, indeed, heal psoriasis.

It soon became apparent to my patients and to me that we were truly on to something. When cases such as these continued to respond favorably, although in varying degrees, we could only conclude that we had been doing something right. The next step for me was to learn all I could about psoriasis from the orthodox, as well as the Cayce, point of view. Armed with the knowledge provided by both schools of thought, I devoted the next decade to treating patients with psoriasis, but only after medical procedures had been exhausted. The results of those years of research follow.

## Does the Regimen Really Work?

This is the question most frequently asked by people seeking answers to this dermatological enigma. My answer is an *emphatic* yes—and no. I am not trying to be cute. It is a fact.

My yes answer applies to most of those patients who seriously commit themselves to the regimen. Of those patients who follow through,

Patient: B.K.
Age: 32 years
Afflicted: 2 years

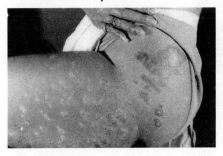

At start of regimen.

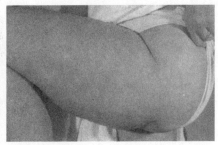

Four months later.

Patient: A.S.
Age: 5 years
Afflicted: 4 years

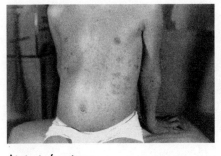

At start of regimen.

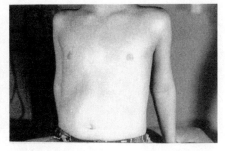

Less than 4 months later.

Patient: E.I.
Age: 8½ years
Afflicted: 1½ years

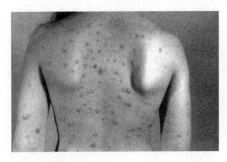

At start of regimen.

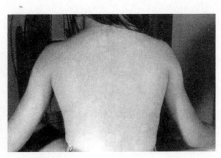

Three months later.

the results can be so outstanding that you would never know they had ever had psoriasis. Perhaps even more important, they rarely, if ever, have to come to me again. This result has often been achieved with children as well.

Those who achieved only moderate results either did not stay with the regimen (they got bored, they began to cheat) or had the attitude, "Okay, I know it works, so I'll stop for now, enjoy whatever I want to eat, and if it flares up again, I'll go back on the diet—eventually." But they rarely did. One thing has been accomplished, however: they are no longer afraid of the disease.

The no side of my answer almost always has its origin in patients' inability or unwillingness to discipline themselves. They want what they want when they want it. That's okay—we all want that. But it is like a star athlete saying, "I want to be the greatest runner in the world, but don't ask me to stop smoking!" It won't happen.

So, the answer to the original question is yes, the regimen works for most people who follow through long enough; no, it doesn't work for those who play at it, do not take it seriously enough, and are always looking for a quick fix.

The real question is not "Does it work?" but "Does the patient work at it?" for therein lies the secret of success—or failure.

## The Way to Go

To the skeptics who proclaim, "This theory has never been proven scientifically," I ask them, what has been? How many people are aware that only 15 to 20 percent of all medical interventions are backed up by scientific studies? This, according to David M. Eddy, MD, PhD, of Duke University, and the U.S. Government Accounting Office, means at least 80 percent are not!

Throughout the long history of healing, cures, benefits, and alleviation of many diseases have taken place without the stamp of approval by a body of scientific experts. If this were not so, the human race would have died off long ago.

My advice to my patients is, just get on with it! View the evidence, meet other patients, and decide for yourself. The scientists will eventually catch up, but in the meantime, you might just get well!

# CHAPTER 3

# About Psoriasis

It never fails to amaze me just how uninformed the average person is about his (or her) skin, especially regarding a psoriatic condition. I can appreciate the fact that most individuals are mainly interested in ridding themselves of the disease without having to delve too deeply into the particular whys and wherefores. More than likely, I, too, would feel much the same way if I suffered from psoriasis. I submit, however, that a person's chances of achieving this goal are greatly enhanced if he is armed with even a smattering of knowledge as to what is actually happening to the skin. Even a minimum of insight and understanding usually instills a desire to approach the prescribed regimen with discipline as well as enthusiasm. Having a physician tell a patient what to do is one thing, but making that patient actually understand the reasoning behind it is even more important. The patient will then do what he is supposed to do and know why he is doing it.

Before I continue to explain this new view and approach to healing psoriasis, I would like to review some known facts about the disease, for my readers to acquire a more thorough understanding of what we are dealing with and the obstacles that we must overcome.

## What Is Psoriasis?

Although the name of the disease is derived from the Greek *psora*, meaning "the itch," itching does not necessarily accompany psoriasis.

When it does, it can be devastating, but in general, I have found that about half of the patients I have cared for were not particularly bothered by an itch.

Eczema, however, another common skin disease, is usually accompanied by an itch. In a later chapter, we will discuss the close link between eczema and psoriasis, which is not ordinarily recognized. It may please the reader to know that once my patients were on the right course, the itch, whether from psoriasis, eczema, or a combination of both, was the first symptom to disappear. This is the first sign that the process is working. It means that there is less surface activity. It then becomes a matter of time and persistence before the scaling stops and the lesions eventually and gradually fade away.

## Your Skin

The skin is a vital, living organ, always moving, changing, teeming with life, and constantly renewing itself. The functions of the skin are numerous, spectacular, and miraculous. Without our being conscious of it, our skin protects us from harmful outside influences, prevents our losing vital internal elements, holds our body together, warns us of potentially harmful internal as well as external temperature changes, plays a major role in our immune system, and performs countless other functions. It also relays pleasurable sensations, beautifies our appearance when cared for, and, in general, equips us with the necessary protective barrier that enables us to live in this world.

That the skin constantly renews itself is an important factor to grasp, for here is where psoriasis enters the picture. Normally, the skin regenerates itself about once a month, or approximately every twenty-eight days. In psoriasis, this process is speeded up; the skin attempts to renew itself every three or four days. One does not have to be a genius to realize that with such a deviation from the norm, something certainly is amiss.

Look at your skin as having two basic layers. The deeper layer, called the *derma* or *dermis,* carries all the blood vessels, nerves, glands, and so forth, and is where new skin cells are formed. The surface layer is called the *epidermis* and is the harder, less delicate, protective component, covering the sensitive structures of the dermis.

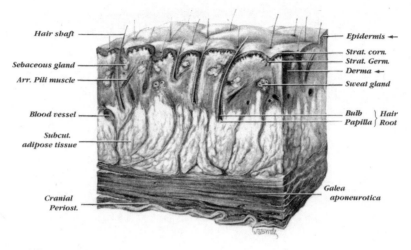

Hair shaft

Sebaceous gland

Arr. Pili muscle

Blood vessel

Subcut. adipose tissue

Cranial Periost.

Epidermis

Strat. corn.
Strat. Germ.
Derma

Sweat gland

Bulb \ Hair
Papilla / Root

Galea aponeurotica

A typical skin section.

Once the dermis forms new skin cells, they begin to migrate outward through various layers to form the cells of the epidermis. It takes about two weeks for these cells to move from the dermis to the epidermal layer. It then takes approximately two more weeks for the cells of the epidermis to die and gradually slough off. In the meantime, new cells have already replaced the old ones. When a person is healthy, this process continues from birth to death, a marvel of biomechanical engineering.

When psoriasis is present, everything goes awry. The dermis tries to produce the new cells at an alarming rate. The surface area becomes red, inflamed, extremely sensitive, visibly raised, and scaly. The specific area involved can rise to three times its thickness above the surface of the epidermis (this is known as *acanthosis*).

## A Comparative View

Upward enlargement of dermal papillae permits up to a threefold increase of the dermoepidermal area, which together with the three-layered germinative cell layer accounts for a ninefold increase in germinative cell population. It is primarily this increase that reduces the turnover time of the epidermis from a normal twenty-eight days to three to four days.

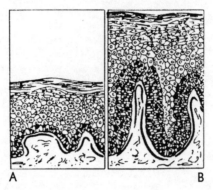

A B

A schematic comparison of normal epidermis (A) and epidermis in psoriasis (B).

A psoriasis victim can form a scale so deep that peeling it off causes bleeding underneath. This is known as the *Auspitz sign*. The cells that are migrating to the surface under these conditions are obviously not normally effective in all of their functions because they have not had enough time to form completely; that is, they are immature. Not only is the process unsightly, but it is unhealthy in that the normal functions of the skin are impaired, rendering the patient prone to internal as well as external environmental hazards.

In spite of all the research carried on since Robert Wilan of England recorded what seems to be the first accurate clinical description of psoriasis, in 1808, the latest statement issued on the subject by the National Institutes of Health (NIH) says, "Scientists do not yet know what causes skin cells to reproduce so rapidly in psoriasis."

To this statement I reply, let's take another look, this time from a different perspective— the inside out, rather than the outside in. From this new approach, we can more readily see why psoriasis lesions form on the surface of the body.

## The Portals of Exit

Continuing to build on what we discussed in chapter 1, we can now go one step further and learn that toxins are emitted from the body via the *perspiratory system* (sweat glands). Why toxins exit more readily from some areas rather than from others is anybody's guess, for sweat glands are everywhere. There are about a hundred such glands in one square centimeter of skin surface, an area about the size of a little fingernail and approximately an eighth of an inch thick.

There is a theory that lesions appear more frequently in areas of the body that are more subject to stress and strain, such as the elbows and the knees. This view, however, does not hold true in all cases, since many people have lesions where there is no particular strain or trauma; for instance, the abdomen or the back.

The most common sites for lesions to form are the scalp, the elbows, the knees, the small of the back, and the lower legs. Lesions can, however, appear literally anywhere, including under toenails and fingernails as well as on the sensitive inner linings of the mucous membranes. Why psoriasis shows itself here, there, or everywhere really is immaterial when it comes to healing the disease.

Specific names have been given to the various types of psoriatic lesions. It must be remembered, however, that regardless of the varying degree of severity or the differences in appearance, the disease is the same. Many people who followed the regimen presented in this book found that different kinds of lesions responded favorably even though they were treated basically the same way. Someone who has had the disease for twenty years cannot realistically expect to respond to treatment as quickly as a person who has had the disease for only two months, although sometimes it is possible. Usually, the longer a person has had the condition, the greater the pollution of the system. Consequently, it will take time to clean out and replenish each cell of the body.

## The Most Common Types of Psoriasis

There are seven common types of psoriasis. They are:

- Common vulgaris
- Guttate
- Flexural
- Generalized/erythrodermic
- Pustular
- Exfoliative
- Psoriatic arthritis

*Common vulgaris* is sometimes referred to as "plaque-type" psoriasis because it looks just as though a plaque has been pasted on the skin—as though it could be simply peeled off. The lesions are often quite noticeably raised, older lesions being darker in color and clearly circumscribed, with adjacent skin uninvolved. Many times, these separated plaques will come together, even during the healing process, and take on a generalized appearance. (See the case of J.R. in the photo section.)

*Guttate* lesions appear as little droplets on small or large areas of the body. Psoriasis often begins with this type in young people between the ages of eight and sixteen. A strep throat frequently precedes the first signs of the disease. Sometimes it will simply clear up by itself, or it can remain and advance to more severe stages. (A question I ask all patients who say their condition seems to have started with a strep throat is whether the psoriasis appeared before or after they started taking antibiotics. This is something to think about.)

*Flexural* psoriasis develops in the natural folds of the skin, such as the armpit, the breast folds, the pubis, the genital area, the groin, and the buttock crease. The area affected appears highly inflamed but lacks scales because of the body's natural lubrication. Since these sections are hardly ever exposed to the sun's rays, and medicated creams can prove most irritating, one can well imagine the joy of accomplishment when these lesions clear up by taking the internal approach I describe.

*Generalized/erythrodermic* psoriasis is widespread, covering most of the body's surface. I have treated cases in which practically every square inch of the skin was affected. The body becomes red all over (*erythro* means "red"), appearing almost like that of boiled lobster. Scaling can be extensive, itching intolerable. If arthritis accompanies the disease, the patient is faced with a double jeopardy. Can this form of psoriasis be healed naturally? It can be and has been, as is evident in the cases of A.M. and L.G. (See the photo section.)

*Pustular* psoriasis is a type in which pus forms on the lesions as it would on boils, indicating an infiltration of white blood cells. (See the case of J.C. in the photo section.) Although rare in itself, it can also become generalized, accompanied by fever and general debility. This is known as *von Zumbusch's disease,* after the physician who first described it. It is most common on the palms of the hands and the soles of the feet. (See the illustrations in chapter 13.)

*Exfoliative* is the most devastating form of psoriasis. The entire skin is involved, and there is profound inflammation and scaling. It may result from an extension or advanced degree of acute guttate or other spreading eruptions. Exfoliative psoriasis usually ends with death in two or three years.

*Psoriatic arthritis* is a form of psoriasis accompanied by an erosive joint disease, sometimes severe, usually involving many joints, particularly the fingers. As the disease advances, demineralization of bone takes place, which is readily discernible on X-ray examinations. Although it strongly resembles rheumatoid arthritis, blood tests reveal the absence of what is called the rheumatoid factor. Psoriatic arthritis is therefore classified as a disease entity in itself. According to Dr. Ronald Marks in his book *Psoriasis,* "Most surveys indicate that one person in twenty with psoriasis has some form of arthritis, and that about one person in twenty with arthritis has some form of psoriasis!"

Age has little to do with this form of psoriasis. Some people develop it in their early teens. It is more prevalent in the twenties or thirties, but middle-aged people are also affected. Because of its importance, I have included a chapter called "The Arthritic Connection" (chapter 16), which deals exclusively with this form of the disease.

Most psoriatics know that the disease is not contagious. This is not very comforting, however, in social or professional interactions when the condition is visible. Because of the disease's physical appearance, it is viewed by the average person as contagious, and contact with the patient is usually avoided, especially by strangers. This can lead to feelings of self-devaluation and embarrassment. Every effort is made to at least "look good"—and for many, that's good enough.

Of course, a person may manifest one type of lesion that will eventually develop into another, or have different types that overlap one another. As previously mentioned, regardless of what form psoriasis takes, it is the same disease, and the treatment is basically the same, with only minor variations. Strange as it may seem, I have seen some severe generalized cases clear up faster than others involving only one or two relatively minor spots. Whatever the extent or type, success was achieved only when the person did not set a time limit but simply followed the prescribed regimen and let nature take its course.

## Statistical Data

Who is, or can be, afflicted with psoriasis? The answer to this question is plain and simple: anyone! Psoriasis does not care about age, race, or gender. There are, however, certain groups in which it is more prevalent. The latest release by the NIH estimates the number of reported psoriatics in the United States alone to be approximately 4 to 6 million, with 150,000 new cases occurring each year. Worldwide, psoriasis afflicts about 2 percent of the population. In Sweden, however, for reasons yet to be determined, the figure is about 3 percent. In Italy and Russia, the psoriasis population is estimated to be as high as 4 percent.

The disease can manifest itself at any time, from infancy (although such cases are rare) to old age. The peak incidence is between the ages of fifteen and thirty-five. Psoriasis appears in both males and females with equal frequency. Dark-skinned people are afflicted less frequently than fair or light-skinned individuals.

John O'Rourke's article in *Let's Live* magazine, "Vitamin A vs. Psoriasis," includes a list called "The Dermatologic Dozen" by Jerome Z. Litt, MD, author of *Your Skin and How to Live in It*. Dr. Litt classifies psoriasis as the fourth most common skin disease, exceeded only by acne, warts, and eczema, in that order. According to George Lewis, MD, there is an associated family history in at least half of all psoriasis cases.

Psoriasis is rare in North and South American Indians. It is common in East African natives and relatively rare in West Africans. It is believed that the reason for the low incidence of psoriasis in African Americans is their ancestral roots in West Africa. Japan is considered a country with a low incidence of the disease, but even there a significant number of citizens are afflicted. In lecturing throughout Japan, I learned that eczema was far more prevalent than psoriasis in that country.

I've often heard that European countries, especially Germany, showed a high incidence of psoriasis just prior to World War II. During the war, the disease practically disappeared when food, especially red meat, was in short supply. After the war, as the economy recovered and the food supply improved, there was a concomitant resurgence of the disease. This in itself tells us something.

In November 1989, I was asked to speak at the First International Conference on Holistic Health and Medicine in Bangalore, India, regarding the research I had conducted on psoriasis. It was the first time that I was able to get an idea of the incidence of psoriasis in the Far East. From the medical doctors who attended my lecture, I learned that psoriasis, eczema, and related skin diseases were widespread not only in India but throughout Southeast Asia. They had a number of patients for me to examine and introduce to this new approach to healing the disease. Based on the 2 percent of the 1 billion people of India who are afflicted with the disease, we can safely assume that there are no less than 20 million psoriatics in India alone. This percentage is likely to be representative of all of Southeast Asia.

Assuming the statisticians are correct, 2 percent of the world's population (estimated at 6.5 billion people) would mean the number of people afflicted with psoriasis throughout the world approaches 100 million! Of particular concern is the fact that psoriasis is on the increase, especially among the young.

The National Psoriasis Foundation (NPF) released the following statistics as they pertain to American psoriasis sufferers:

- 6.4 million Americans are affected.
- It is slightly more prevalent in women than in men.
- The average age of sufferers is twenty-eight, but psoriasis is seen from birth to age ninety.
- Children under the age of ten constitute 10 to 15 percent of sufferers.
- Psoriatic arthritis affects 10 to 20 percent of psoriasis sufferers.
- From 150,000 to 260,000 new cases are reported each year.
- The annual outlay of outpatient costs is $1.6 to $3.2 billion.
- Four hundred people with psoriasis are granted Social Security disabilities each year.
- Annually, approximately 400 people die of psoriasis-related causes.
- Over 1.5 million people per year are seen by U.S. physicians for psoriasis.

## Mechanisms That Trigger Psoriasis

Usually, a victim of psoriasis first notices a small sore somewhere on the body, a sore that doesn't heal. It just seems to get worse and begins to spread. More sores then erupt in different areas. Some of the sores remain small or eventually disappear, but in most instances, they get worse as time goes on, and the patient begins to seek relief.

There are occasions when the first signs of the disease appear after an injury or an abrasion of the skin. The damaged area does not heal properly and psoriatic lesions begin to develop along the site of the injury. This is known as the *Koebner phenomenon.* Vigorous scrubbing, scratching, or picking at the area only makes it worse. Low humidity, systemically administered drugs, and severe emotional stress can also be triggering factors preceding the first outbreak of the disease. Even using a loofah sponge instead of a soft cloth or just your hands while showering can irritate the skin to the point of severe inflammation.

There are many cases in which a pregnant woman with psoriasis seemingly improves during the gestation period. However, the disease usually returns after she delivers.

The fact is that the body is prone to being psoriatic long before the first signs of the disease appear, because internal pollution, the major causative factor of the disease, first affects the body on the *inside.*

## Are Psoriatics Healthy? A Personal Comment

Because psoriasis is rarely considered to be life threatening, it is often thought of by the scientific community as less important than other, devastating diseases. In fact, one expert in the field of psoriasis research refers to most psoriatics as basically healthy people with a skin problem. I view this as a contradiction in terms. A psoriatic condition is the first sign that a patient is not in a healthy state.

One of my patients who had lesions on every square inch of his body said to me, "Doctor, I don't understand it. I am a healthy man— but look at me, I'm a mess!" And a mess he was—for twenty-five years. I am convinced that the word *healthy* is a total misnomer in a case like this. When discomfort, soreness, itching, cracking of the skin, and so forth accompanies psoriasis, that patient indeed feels sick and unhealthy. I have had patients with massive lesions all over their bodies, but without discomfort, who looked at their condition quite objectively and unemotionally. For some reason, they were spared the painful irritation that often accompanies the disease.

In other words, when there are no perpetually distressing symptoms, it is not difficult for some people to live with this illness. When a patient is faced with irritating symptoms day in and day out, he or she is more inclined to seek relief by whatever means possible. But in either case, the patient is equally unhealthy and equally in need of treatment.

## Therapies Are Available

The list of therapeutic measures developed over the years is long and varied. Such measures encompass *topical* (external) therapy, *systemic* (internal) therapy, and *dual* therapy such as photochemotherapy (a combination of a drug with ultraviolet [UV] light). The results of the procedures also vary. With some patients, they are often quite encouraging, whereas with others, the response can be disastrous. As with other treatments, some people respond favorably; others do not. Practically every orthodox procedure involves some form of external application, usually in the form of salves, creams, and lotions, but techniques ranging from tar baths to photochemotherapy to laser beams have been applied, again with varying degrees of success or failure. Ultrasound is experimentally used in some cases, as well as simple adhesive tape. Fluorinated steroids, steroid injections, and glucocorticosteroids (steroid compounds) are often used, but with careful monitoring, as the possible harmful side effects, including thinning skin and redness and dilation of surface blood vessels, are well known.

The *Goeckerman regimen* is one of the oldest and most effective therapies and is named after the American doctor who devised it. Discovered over sixty years ago, the regimen consists of applying distilled tar, crude or refined, to the skin, leaving it on overnight in most cases, and irradiating the skin the next morning with UV rays. Many times, this procedure clears the skin for long periods of time, but the mess involved is a disadvantage to the patient. This method is used to this day as it has been proven to be moderately safe and effective.

*PUVA (psoralen ultraviolet light type A)* refers to photochemotherapy. This type of therapy has been used experimentally for several years at Massachusetts General Hospital. It is the combination of a drug, psoralen, taken orally and followed in about two hours by carefully controlled exposure to UV light–type A therapy. Psoralen causes the skin to become more sensitive to the absorption of UV light. PUVA, although approved by the Food and Drug Administration (FDA) in May 1982, has possible serious side effects such as the development of certain forms of skin cancer, cataract formation, and an actual burn from the lights themselves. For these and other reasons, researchers use this form of therapy only in severe cases and urge restraint in the long-term use of PUVA treatment.

*Dialysis of the blood* (hemodialysis) is a treatment used to purify the blood of people with chronic kidney disease. However, it has been found to help in cases of severe psoriasis, but again, the long-term effects are not yet known. It is used only as a last-resort procedure.

*Aromatic retinoid* is a drug chemically related to vitamin A. It is a synthetic form of vitamin A, remarkably effective in some severe cases. It should, however, be prescribed with care because, according to the NIH, high doses can cause inflammation of the lips, hair loss, and abnormal dryness of the eyes, skin, and mouth.

*Ultraviolet light—type A* (UVA) by itself is not the best method of choice for clearing psoriasis. As mentioned earlier, when it is used extensively, it could have serious side effects. This type should be applied only in a dermatologist's office or a hospital setting.

*Ultraviolet light—type B* (UVB) is the most widely used light in the treatment of psoriasis and has been used for over fifty years. A patient must build up a tolerance for it. Consequently, at first, small doses are applied for about thirty seconds and gradually increased. The effects are practically the same as with normal sunlight. UVB light does not penetrate the skin as deeply as UVA.

*Methotrexate* (MTX), a cancer drug, is often used internally on the most severe cases. Liver biopsies, however, are routinely conducted on patients using MTX, because after prolonged use, the drug is known to have harmful effects on the internal (visceral) structures of the body, particularly the liver.

*Activated vitamin D cream,* according to Dr. Michael Holick, MD, the director of the Clinical Research Center at Boston University School of Medicine, has been quite favorably used by a significant number of psoriasis cases. There is also an oral form of activated vitamin D, but it might not be as effective as the topical form.

The list of standard external salves, such as anthralin (dithranol), PsoriGel, Estar, salicylic acid combined with coal tar or steroid cream, Diprosone, and so forth, is too long to mention. They all have their advantages and disadvantages, but whatever the methods used, they are palliative at best, masking the symptoms of an elusive disease that appears on the surface but originates elsewhere in the body.

*Treatment at the Dead Sea.* Lying in the deepest fault in the Earth's crust in Israel is the body of water known as the Dead Sea. Because of its extremely high salt content (nine times saltier than the oceans), nothing can live in it, thus the name "Dead" Sea. For centuries, those who could afford it traveled to the Dead Sea for cosmetic and health reasons, claiming its waters cured psoriasis as well as arthritis and rheumatism.

Because the Dead Sea is twelve hundred feet below sea level, there is a longer column of air through which solar radiation must travel. This filters out much of the UVB light, leaving a higher amount of UVA light to which one is exposed, says Dr. Brian Diffey, principal physician, at Dryburn Hospital in Durham, England. "However," he adds, "a person must sunbathe eight hours a day for three to four weeks at the Dead Sea to achieve clearance."

Also included as part of the therapeutic regimen is soaking in the Dead Sea, which may include various emollients and moisturizers that soften and peel heavy plaque-type psoriasis. In addition, it is believed that rest from the patient's stressful daily living and psychological group therapy aid in its effectiveness. Although medical authorities question the true value of the Dead Sea, tourists continue their pilgrimage there for health reasons.

*Cyclosporine,* a relatively new systemic treatment, was first noted to be effective in cases of psoriatic arthritis and psoriasis in 1979. The *New England Journal of Medicine* (January 31, 1991, 324 no.5) released a paper by Charles Ellis on the effect cyclosporine has on severe plaque-type psoriasis. There are, however, reservations as to its continued use, because it has been suggested that long-term use of cyclosporine may lead to suppression of the natural immune system and systemic tumor (lymphoma) formations and because of the potential toxicity of the drug. The journal reports, "Thus, although cyclosporine is a highly effective agent for severe psoriasis, it should probably be used only as short-term therapy until more experience is reported."

## The T-Cell Theory

T-cells, also known as killer cells, form the body's first line of defense against foreign invaders and antigens of one sort or another. Without them you would be defenseless.

In 1995, researchers at Rockefeller University discovered that T-cells are found in large numbers at the sites of psoriatic lesions. They concluded that since the T-cells are concentrated in such numbers, they must be the cause of the disease. Therefore, the logical thing to do is to destroy the T-cells and thereby destroy the disease. Studies were done to develop an injectable drug that would seek and destroy the T-cells, which would theoretically conquer the disease. The list of prescribed systemic medications is extensive, but at the time of this writing, perhaps the most common ones are Amevive, Embrel, and Raptiva.

## Further Information

Presently, there are a number of newly developed medications available to the psoriatic and/or psoriatic arthritic patients that require a medical doctor's prescription.

For a more extensive treatise on the subject of over-the-counter products and prescription items, contact the National Psoriasis Foundation, 6600 SW 92nd Avenue, Suite 300, Portland, OR 97223, 1-800-723-9166, or online at www.psoriasis.org, and ask for their "Psoriasis and Psoriatic Arthritis Treatment Guide, 2004/2005."

## There Is Another Way

Surprisingly, most of my patients are quick to accept the idea that psoriasis is essentially an internal malfunction. Once this is explained, their reaction is, "It makes sense!" Rarely, if ever, have I met with resistance from a patient concerning the theory that psoriasis is due to internal pollution making its way through the skin. This is especially convincing after presenting patients with tangible evidence of healing. For the first time since becoming afflicted, they are given an explanation for their skin disorder that they can understand.

Armed with this newfound knowledge, those patients who are open to it are ready to proceed—this time, however, their attack on the problem will be launched from a different direction: a natural alternative.

# CHAPTER 4

# The Natural Alternative

There is a simple, twofold premise on which this alternative approach to healing psoriasis is based:

1. Clear out the poisons that have accumulated in the body.
2. Prevent further intake of toxic elements.

I say, without reservation, that once these two processes are set in motion, regeneration begins, and new skin forms to replace the old.

## The Cayce/Pagano Regimen

Perhaps my readers will view the prior statement as rather bold, but I can attest to the fact that this is exactly what happens. The previous chapter explained how new cells constantly form in the dermal layer of our skin and migrate to the outer layer to form the epidermis, which then sloughs off. This is an established scientific fact. Therefore, it is not inappropriate to say a "new" skin forms; it happens naturally, every month. The psoriatic's aim is to ensure that next time, it will be new skin without the addition of toxic elements.

How long it will take for an individual to detoxify is impossible to determine. Each person has his or her own built-in time clock. However, the fastest responding severe case that I have ever treated took thirty days to clear, after suffering for thirty years; the longest case took two years after suffering for twenty-eight years. Keep in mind that it is the *direction* and not the *speed* that counts in this approach.

To achieve the two basic requirements stated at the beginning of this chapter, the following measures are essential:

1. Internal cleansing
2. A high alkaline–low acidic diet
3. Specific herbal teas
4. Adjustments of the spine
5. External applications
6. Right thinking—a *must* in the healing of any disease

As we proceed, all of these measures will be dealt with separately. Since each individual is different, certain measures will have more significance to some people than to others. Here is where the skill and sensitivity of the physician, or the patient's own personal perceptions, come into play. In this way, the patient is able to determine his or her own strengths and weaknesses and proceed accordingly.

It will soon become obvious that this regimen makes you cognizant not only of your skin, but of your body as a whole. All of the organs or systems of the body are dependent on one another. This is why something that benefits one system automatically benefits another, and conversely, something that breaks down one system can break down another. When all of these systems function properly, the body eventually reaches a state of equilibrium, or homeostasis, becoming a full-fledged working unit of energy—the natural state of health.

## Holistic Healing

Holism, or holistic healing, has become a household word. Mankind has come to the point of realizing that many things seen on the outside are actually formed or caused by things that are unseen. In considering holistic healing, it is essential to recognize the human being as a unity of spirit, mind, and body. It is the proper balancing of these three aspects that constitutes the health and well-being of the individual.

Plato remarked in the *Phaedrus,* "For this is the great error of our day in the treatment of the human body, that the physicians separate the soul from the body." Recently, many physicians have come to the same conclusion.

For instance, a skin disease may originate in an emotional upset such as harbored resentment and remain with a person until the cause of the resentment is understood or eradicated. A headache has often been traced to a forgotten injury to the tailbone or to digestive disturbances caused by a poor diet. Improper absorption and assimilation of certain trace minerals can be the cause of mental illness, including some forms of schizophrenia.

The Cayce material continually emphasizes the triune approach to health that encourages the balance of all three forces—spirit, mind, and body—as mandatory for our health and happiness, which is our birthright. This triune principle is the cornerstone of my research. In essence, it is properly setting in motion the forces of nature within the individual that will help the body heal itself.

## There Are Times

There are all degrees of flare-ups that may occur during the healing process. Some are mild, whereas others can be severe. Usually flare-ups are relatively mild, and people get through them easily. Once the breakthrough of new skin begins to show itself, total renewal of the skin eventually occurs.

There are times, however, for some sufferers, when the flare-up becomes so terrifying that medical intervention is warranted. Usually, small doses of methotrexate (MTX) are administered by a dermatologist, which helps calm the skin down and gets the patient through what is called the purge period, the healing crisis, or, scientifically speaking, the "Herxheimer reaction." In the past few years, I have seen it happen only two or three times. Most people want to remain on the regimen and follow through. With the guidance of their medical doctor, they can gradually cut down on the MTX, until it can be eliminated altogether. It is a matter of getting through the rough periods when the skin takes on a rebellious attitude. Recognize it for what it is: the body purging itself, throwing off toxins that have been locked in for so many years. It's as though the disease is not going to give up without a fight.

Does the MTX work every time? No. Does it work often? Yes. It is at such times, when the MTX works, that the *natural alternative* (sometimes referred to as the Cayce/Pagano regimen), combined with medicine, can bring about a most gratifying result.

## The "1-2-3" Concept of the Disease

The results obtained over thirty-five years of studying, observing, and being actively engaged in the clinical management of psoriasis have led me to formulate what I call the "1-2-3" concept of the disease.

1. Psoriasis is the external manifestation of the body's attempt to eliminate accumulated toxins that have invaded the lymphatics, bloodstream, and body cells primarily through thin or porous intestinal walls.

2. Psoriasis is characterized by inflamed patches (lesions) with silvery scales of skin that slough off in three to four days instead of the normal twenty-eight-day period.

3. Psoriasis is alleviated, controlled, or even possibly cured by taking the necessary steps to heal the intestinal walls and by opening up the normal channels of elimination, as well as preventing further toxins from entering the system.

In the chapters that follow, I will help you further understand the basics of the disease from this new perspective. This will lead to viewing the healing of psoriasis as a process rather than a condition dependent on a particular commodity—a process I call the *natural alternative*.

# CHAPTER 5

# Internal Cleansing

W hat better place to begin our healing process than at the very beginning? Common sense tells us to "clean house" before redecorating. In the case of psoriasis, the first condition to correct is the accumulated pollution that has infected the entire bloodstream and, subsequently, all the organs and cells of the body. This is accomplished by opening up the normal channels of elimination, primarily the bowels and the kidneys and, secondarily, the skin and the lungs.

Obviously, the most effective cleansing is obtained by clearing out the bowels and the kidneys. This releases the backup pressure on the liver and gall ducts as well as the intestines, allowing free passage of their waste accumulations. In this way, the hepatic (liver) cells are free to perform one of their most important tasks: filtering out and purifying the blood and lymph.

Chronic constipation and poor eliminative habits are the major causes of colon impaction, which, in itself, is one of the main reasons for the breakdown of the intestinal walls. In his classic medical textbook, *Symptoms of Visceral Disease,* Francis M. Pottenger, MD, a world-renowned authority on neurology, clearly explains the effect a sluggish bowel has on the intestinal wall: "When the contents of the intestinal tract are delayed in their movement through the intestine, they undergo certain changes, which are more or less irritating and injurious to the intestinal wall. Stasis from this cause is usually accompanied by the absorption of toxins."

# The Colon (Large Intestine)

It is impossible to overemphasize the importance of paying close attention to the colon and its proper functioning.

Certain physical abnormalities can cause a malfunction of the colon. Even if there is no pathological process such as a tumor formation or stricture, the colon, in some people, may be excessively lengthened beyond its normal five feet in the average adult. This is called a redundant colon. Its positioning in the abdominal cavity may also be abnormal, causing an irregular twist or turn that slows down the normal passage of fecal matter.

The illustrations on pages 38, 39, and 40 show a few of the more common abnormal conditions that may occur in the colon. They are reproduced here through the courtesy of Dr. Bernard Jensen, from his book, *Tissue Cleansing through Bowel Management.*

In other words, there can be anatomical reasons for malfunction of the colon; it is not always a matter of poor diet or bad toilet habits. Whatever the reason for a malfunction, if at all possible, steps should

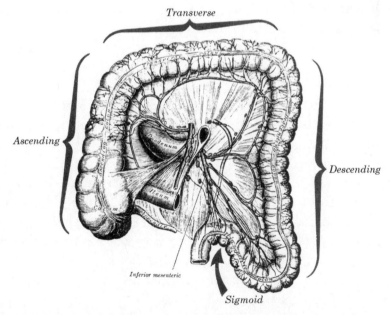

The colon is divided into 4 parts: ascending, transverse, descending, and sigmoid.

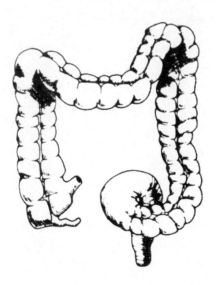 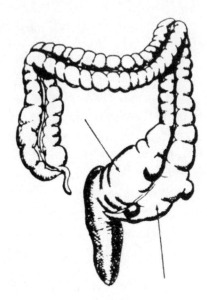

*Normal Colon*                *Ballooned Sigmoid*

be taken to correct it. Fortunately, anatomical abnormalities are found in only a minority of cases. More often than not, the culprit in psoriasis is improper elimination due to poor eating habits, which, in most cases, can be corrected. Both require discipline on the patient's part. With regard to eating, the patient should select easily digestible and more absorbable types of foods. (Diet is dealt with quite thoroughly in chapter 6 and appendix A.)

Poor toilet habits are more common than may be ordinarily suspected. It is amazing to discover what some people consider normal. For instance, one patient, when asked about the frequency of his bowel movements, replied, "Oh, Doc! I have no problem there. I go once every four or five days without fail!" Can you imagine the look of surprise on his face when I explained to him that having "no problem" meant eliminating once, twice, or even three times each day? He had labored under a misconception for many years because a physician once told him that infrequent elimination was nothing to be concerned about, and, in his case, it was normal. Once his bowels were regulated to eliminating every day, his psoriasis, as well as other health problems

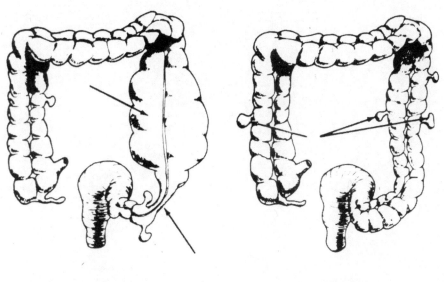

**Colitis**                              **Diverticula**

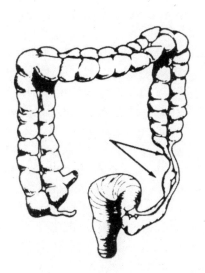 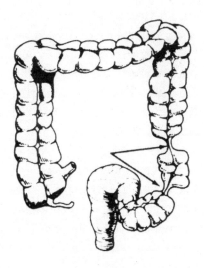

**Spasm**                                **Stricture**

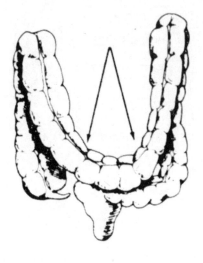

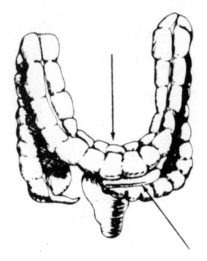

*Prolapsus*

*Prolapsus with pressure on lower organs*

that he faced, disappeared. Since then (eight years ago), he has never had a recurrence of his symptoms.

The reason another patient of mine did not eliminate more than once a week was, to quote her, "I didn't like going to the bathroom!" I eventually learned that this was a habit shared by all members of her family. She had actually been raised to believe that defecating was something dirty and should be done only when absolutely necessary.

Once this patient was convinced of the fallacy of this idea, she made it a point to alter her habits. In time, good results were evident in that her generalized psoriatic condition showed a gradual improvement. During one of the meetings of psoriasis patients I held in my office, she remarked to other patients that she had not realized the beneficial effect that regular bowel movements would have on her skin.

The principle to grasp here is that blockages or partial blockages of the colon, for whatever reason, are detrimental to the general well-being of the individual. The result of such impairments may vary considerably, taking the form of one disease or another.

Categorically speaking, rheumatoid arthritis, eczema, scleroderma, lupus erythematosus, psoriasis, and a number of other systemic diseases may very well have the same basic cause. The course of treatment is, therefore, essentially the same if the patient chooses the alternative route explained in this book. In these types of diseases, therapy should begin with internal cleansing, regardless of which disease it is. When this procedure is followed, the body can concentrate its efforts on rebuilding more quickly than if it had to destroy the "enemy"—that is, the accumulated toxins—before starting reconstruction. It follows, then, that the more effective the internal cleansing, the quicker the disappearance of psoriasis.

## The Kidneys

The kidneys play as important a role in ridding the body of toxins as do the liver and the bowel. They do so by filtering potentially dangerous impurities out of the blood and discarding them daily through the bladder in the form of urine. Each hour, the blood filters through the kidneys twice. Vitamins, amino acids, glucose, hormones, and so forth are returned to the bloodstream, the excess residue eliminated in the urine. The end product of protein is *urea.* It is vital that the kidneys keep the level of urea in balance. If there is too little of it in the blood, it can indicate that the liver is not functioning properly; if there is too much present, uremic poisoning of the blood can ensue, jeopardizing a person's life.

The kidneys also have many other functions, such as helping in the production of red blood cells, maintaining normal chemistry levels of the cells, and playing a distinctive role in the acid-alkaline balance, a topic of utmost concern to the psoriatic.

Is it any wonder that the kidneys have been referred to often as the "master chemists" of the body? Keeping your kidneys cleansed and free of accumulated waste is accomplished principally by drinking an adequate amount of pure water daily. Six to eight glasses of water each day, in addition to all other liquids, is recommended. I often advocate that a patient keep a gallon of pure mountain-spring water in the refrigerator at all times, and if desired, add the juice of a few fresh limes or lemons. This is not only a thirst-quenching drink, but it also helps flush the kidneys and is alkaline-reacting. In the next chapter, we will discuss the significance of alkaline- versus acid-reacting food and drink and how this relates to psoriasis. In recent years, the condition of urinary incontinence (loss of bladder control) has become more recognized as a problem that affects 10 million people in this country, mostly women. If people with this condition also have psoriasis, they are faced with another problem, since following the recommendation to drink six to eight glasses of water daily could make life unbearable. Fortunately, there are medical procedures that have proven to be very effective, even curative. If a patient suffers from urinary incontinence, I highly recommend that she or he have it corrected medically before proceeding with this regimen.

Dialysis, which is mentioned in chapter 3, is a medical procedure that filters out impurities in the blood of patients whose kidneys no longer function properly. An interesting phenomenon has been observed in some kidney patients on dialysis who also have psoriasis. They show a marked improvement in their skin while undergoing this treatment. Since the sole purpose of this medical procedure is to purify the blood, I think it is quite significant to note that the skin reacts in such a positive way when dialysis is administered. This interesting reaction was accidentally discovered years ago. Today, dialysis therapy is used on a limited basis, and only as a last resort, in extremely severe cases of psoriasis.

This indicates that properly functioning kidneys play a significant role in keeping the skin free of blemishes.

## The Skin and the Lungs

The average person rarely recognizes the skin and lungs as avenues of escape for toxins and impurities. In fact, they are the secondary organs of elimination—second only to the bowel and the kidneys. It is when we consider this function of the skin that we begin to recognize the reason for psoriatic lesions, as well as the irritating, rashlike manifestation of eczema and other skin abnormalities.

### The Skin

An illustration showing a typical skin section appears in chapter 3, where the sweat glands are discussed in regard to their function as portals of exit for accumulated toxins, thus fulfilling a major purpose of the skin. Did you know, however, that within that same ⅛-inch square segment of skin there are not only one hundred sweat glands, but also twelve feet of nerves, hundreds of nerve endings, ten hair follicles, fifteen sebaceous glands, and three feet of blood vessels?

In the eighteen square feet of skin that covers the body, there are about 2 million sweat glands. Each one is a tiny tightly coiled fifty-inch tube buried deep in the dermis and rising out of it, as a duct to the surface. In total, there are six miles of these ducts. These sweat glands function almost continually, extracting water, salt, and waste from the blood. Is it any wonder that the skin is the largest organ in the body?

## The Lungs

Most people fail to appreciate the role the lungs play in the removal of internal toxins. The specific function of the lungs is to take air from the external environment, oxygenate the blood to be distributed throughout every body cell, and remove gaseous poisons, particularly carbon dioxide, from the body. Deep-breathing exercises such as those taught in yoga have proven how pure air, properly inhaled, retained for a short time, and exhaled slowly, greatly improves the physical and mental health of an individual.

In a normal state of health, one is hardly cognizant of the lungs. Indeed, it has been said that when you are aware of your lungs, you are already in trouble!

In a stationary person, the lungs normally pump in and out about seventeen times a minute. Walking requires more oxygen, so the pumping increases to approximately twenty-four breaths per minute. Running doubles that amount to about fifty breaths. When exercise is conducted in the open air, the blood's used gases are expelled and replaced by oxygen more freely; hence, exposing the lungs to impurities such as chemical fumes and automotive exhaust should be avoided as much as possible. The psoriatic should be aware of these facts and act accordingly, for by purifying the lung fields, a major step is taken to rid the body of psoriasis.

Take care of your lungs. Nurture them by supplying them with the fresh air they need to function properly. They will, in turn, take care of every cell, organ, and muscle in your body, supplying you with oxygen for every activity, from sleeping to running to thinking. Guard these sentinels of vital energy well, for your lungs truly provide you with the breath of life.

## The Liver

The liver is so remarkable an organ that some cultures regard it as the site of life. One cannot begin to understand how the body filters out toxic elements, without an appreciation of the incredible task carried out by the liver. When the liver is not functioning properly, not only do toxins build up in the body, but changes in mood, behavior, and general health can occur. It has been determined that the liver is responsible for over five hundred separate activities. Of these various functions, the ones we are most concerned with are the breakdown and excretion of poisonous materials. The liver is one of the major filtering glands of the body. Its many functions are primarily carried out by a single, remarkable structural unit called the *hepatic cell*. There are approximately 300 billion of these unique cells in one liver, which, among other things, filter two and one-half pints of blood per minute when the body is at rest. In one year, it amounts to filtering out enough blood to fill twenty-three milk trucks! The liver has remarkable regenerative powers as well. If 90 percent of the liver were removed, the remaining piece could still function. In fact, it might even grow back to its original size.

As miraculous as the liver is in its makeup and functions, it can nevertheless reach a breaking point as a result of constant abuse and overtaxation. Barring direct injury to this organ and/or pathological processes, the most common reason for liver depletion is improper diet or liquid intake. When the liver becomes too seriously overtaxed with the resulting toxins, a breakdown of hepatic cells occurs, thereby opening the door to malfunction, infection, and congestion.

Fortunately, the liver has incredible regenerative powers when given the right fuel to work with. It behooves us, therefore, to do all in our power to keep this vital organ pliable and free of accumulated toxins. One of the most obvious ways of accomplishing this is to prevent destructive food items from entering the system at all, hence the importance of proper nutrition. We do well to eat or drink items that

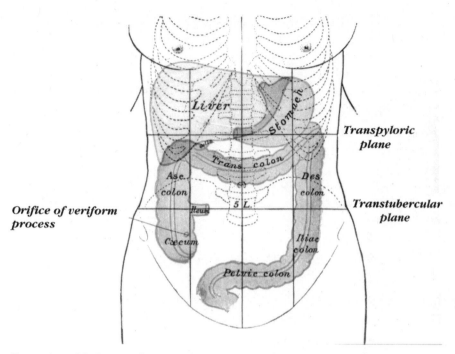

The position of the liver in relation to other structures of the abdominal viscera.

have a known internal cleansing effect, such as those recommended in chapter 6 and appendix A, which deal with diet and nutrition.

An effective external measure to help regenerate the liver is to gently but thoroughly massage the entire liver area with an olive–peanut oil mixture, unless one has an allergy to peanuts.

Another effective procedure I suggest to some patients is the application of warm castor oil packs directly over the liver. The simplest way to accomplish this is to saturate the liver area with castor oil; place a warm, damp, soft cloth (preferably white flannel, four layers thick) over the area; then cover with a piece of plastic wrap. A heating pad, set at medium, is placed over the entire pack for one to two hours. I have found, to my satisfaction, that massaging the liver or applying hot castor oil packs to it are among the healthiest measures that can be taken to help this organ perform its function of purifying the blood.

I advise all my patients to use discretion when using these hot packs. Some people's skin can be more sensitive than that of others.

## The Liver/Skin–Kidney/Lung Correlation

Many theories have been put forward as to the effect internal pollution has on the body, but when it comes to skin and lung disorders, none can compare with the work of Henry G. Bieler, MD, in his excellent book, *Food Is Your Best Medicine.* I suggest that you carefully read the following passage from his book, for it provides the basic information needed for an understanding of the liver/skin–kidney/lung connection:

> The liver and the kidneys are important eliminative organs. For the liver, the natural avenue of elimination, of course, is through the bowel; for the kidneys, through the bladder and urethra.
>
> However, when the liver is congested and cannot perform its eliminative function, waste matter (toxins) is thrown into the bloodstream. Similarly, when the kidneys are inflamed, toxins are also dammed up in the blood. Toxic blood must discharge its toxins or the person dies, so nature uses vicarious avenues of elimination or substitutes. The lungs, therefore, will take over the task of eliminating some of the wastes that should have gone through the kidneys, or the skin will take over for the liver. It stands to reason that the lungs do not make very good kidneys. From the irritation caused by the elimination of poison through this "vicarious" channel, we can get bronchitis, pneumonia, or tuberculosis, as is determined by the particular chemistry of the poison being eliminated. Thus, we can say that the lungs are acting vicariously for the kidneys or are being called into play, under duress, as substitute kidneys. In the same way, if the bile poisons in the blood come out through the skin, we get the various irritations of the skin, resulting in the many skin diseases, or through the mucous membranes (inside skin) as the various catarrhs, or through the skin as boils, carbuncles, acne, etc. Thus, the skin is substituting for the liver or a vicarious elimination is occurring through the skin.

Clearly, one part of the body cannot be separated from another. All the organs are interconnected. Polluting one area spills over to pollute another; conversely, by purifying one area, you purify another.

The proper goal for psoriatics is to purify the entire system. When this is accomplished, no matter how long it takes, the inner condition of cleansed body cells will be reflected in the outer appearance of the body's surface—a healthy-looking skin.

## Toxins

Since toxic buildup is what actually causes psoriasis, it will do no harm for the psoriatic to learn about the meaning of the word *toxin*. If nothing else, you will at least be able to identify the enemy.

To begin with, a toxin is a poisonous substance derived from animal or vegetable cells. When toxins invade the bloodstream, the result is *toxemia,* a condition in which the blood contains an overabundance of poisons. Toxins are produced by body cells or by the growth of microorganisms, which cause a general infection whereby the blood contains toxins but not bacteria. When the buildup becomes too much for the body's natural defense mechanism to handle, the patient is considered toxic. Symptoms such as tiredness, malaise, lack of energy, and often halitosis (bad breath) are common signs of toxicity.

Why is it important that the psoriatic understand what toxemia is? Francis Pottenger, MD, states that "in all cases of toxemia, and particularly those of acute toxemia, we find a tendency to *sluggishness of action in the gastrointestinal tract*" (emphasis added). Obviously, when this "sluggishness" occurs, there is a greater tendency for reabsorbing toxic elements through the walls of both the small and the large intestines. It is my contention that this is the major cause of most degenerative, debilitating diseases, as well as various skin conditions, including psoriasis.

### Improved Bathroom Facilities

Since the beginning of the twentieth century, man's life span has doubled. Most of us presume that this is due to advances in medical technology, wonder drugs, surgical procedures, and so forth. Undoubtedly, these have contributed greatly to man's longevity. Seldom recognized, however, is the role that improved sanitary conditions play, especially the advent of indoor plumbing. A new era of health and longevity began when toilet facilities within the home became common.

Today, such accommodations are taken for granted, especially by young people. In years gone by, the outhouse was recognized as the cubicle of privacy. As it was located at least several yards away from the main house, it involved extra effort to visit, especially in the dead of winter. The tendency was to wait, avoiding evacuation until absolutely necessary. On occasion, it would be days before a person relieved himself. This naturally caused a backup pressure of fecal matter, which often was allowed to reach a point of autointoxication and unquestionably acted as a precursor of many systemic diseases. Evidence of this is found in comparing our present-day life span of eighty years or so with the average of about forty years at the turn of the twentieth century. It is no longer necessary to retain all the poisons and waste matter because of uncomfortable, inconvenient toilet facilities, for indoor plumbing provides relief but a few steps away in the comfort of your own home.

## The "Glut" Response

Toxins form not only from substances known to be detrimental to the body but from those that may become toxic if overindulged in. Ordinarily, such foods may not have a deleterious effect, but because of an insatiable desire for a particular food, some people have a tendency to gorge themselves. This causes what I call a "glut" response. In these cases, a chemical imbalance is bound to occur, and the body will respond by producing skin conditions, allergic reactions, glandular dysfunctions, and myriad other ailments.

## Thoughts and Toxins

As previously emphasized, clearing the body of accumulated toxins is of the utmost importance. Just as significant, however, is the maintenance of a healthy mental attitude. Have no doubt about it: negative, destructive thoughts also produce acidic toxins that can do still more harm to an already polluted system.

For instance, you cannot have continued feelings of hatred without developing stomach or liver problems. Negative emotions such as uncontrollable anger or jealousy can cause digestive or heart disorders. Animosity and worrying can lead only to further distressful systemic conditions. Thoughts most assuredly affect the internal environment of the body. This is now fully accepted and recognized by the scientific community.

You should learn to recognize and appreciate the cheerful aspects of life and avoid negative situations and personalities, referred to colloquially as "real downers." A sunny, smiling countenance goes a long way, not only for yourself but for those around you. This important subject matter is further discussed in chapters 10 and 11.

To summarize, the goal is to rid the body of toxins that have accumulated over a long period of time and avoid reintroducing more of those same toxic elements to the system. Learn to recognize the pollutants, usually certain foods, and avoid them at all costs. We start the entire process with internal cleansing.

## Effective Cleansing Measures

Since the primary organs of elimination are the bowels and the kidneys, it is important to concentrate on their proper functioning and the measures that will help to purify them. The effectiveness of the diet, teas, adjustments, oils, and so forth will increase a hundredfold if the body is kept internally cleansed. By doing so, one begins fresh, renewing the body even down to the cellular level. In my opinion, the initial cleansing is the turning point in psoriasis—the point when the disease process begins to reverse itself. As soon as body pollutants are no longer assimilated and a cleansing diet is followed, detoxification begins to take place.

As purification takes hold, more and more toxins exit every cell in the body. When this stage is reached, nutritious food elements are assimilated properly, and the rebuilding begins on a cellular level. It is only a matter of time before complete renewal occurs.

The toxins produced by the body "sludge" are removed primarily by ingesting laxative foods and drinks and by cleansing the large intestine. In addition, perspiration induced by taking a steam bath, coupled with deep-breathing exercises, is also beneficial in removing toxic elements from the skin itself and also from the lung fields. An adequate daily intake of pure water will help to ensure kidney purification. In this way, the body rids itself of accumulated toxins. For greater effectiveness, a colonic irrigation or home enema should be preceded by a cleansing diet, several of which will be discussed later in this chapter.

## The High Colonic Irrigation

With regard to the bowel (colon), there is, in my opinion, no more effective cleansing measure devised by modern man than the high *colonic irrigation,* or high enema. It is best described as a gentle, effective method of hydrotherapy used to cleanse the large intestine. The high colonic cleans out the sigmoid, descending, transverse, and ascending colon, which, in total, measures approximately five feet in the average adult. Fecal matter and waste can accumulate over a period of years around the inner lining and convolutions of the colon. Since numerous lymphatics are directly attached to the outer walls of the colon, toxic matter constantly feeds the lymphatic attachments and invades the lymphatic chain. A properly administered high colonic irrigation is capable of flushing out impacted waste matter that has adhered to the inner walls of the large intestine. Once this is accomplished, the impurities will have been flushed out; consequently, the "seepage" of toxins will no longer occur.

The ultimate benefit is that this relieves the tendency toward chronic constipation, thereby aiding in preventing intestinal stasis (an undue delay in the passage of fecal matter along the intestines), which was referred to earlier in the quotation from Francis M. Pottenger.

A properly administered high colonic can often mean the difference between success and failure for the psoriatic. I stress "properly administered" because a good technician, experienced in high colonic therapy, is not easy to find, and the sanitary conditions of the unit itself are as important as the technique applied. It is of the utmost importance that strict sanitary conditions prevail wherever colonics are administered. Even though the bowel may not be considered a sterile area, it should be cleansed with sterile equipment to avoid contamination. If the therapist who administers the colonic, usually a registered nurse, is reputable and maintains his or her equipment according to strict professional requirements, there should be no problem. If a patient feels apprehensive about either the condition or the appearance of the unit or the qualifications of the technician, I advise him to excuse himself under the guise that he will have to give it more thought. I advise that he not return if there is any question about the professionalism of the technician or the sanitary condition of the unit.

In recent years, disposable nozzles and hoses have become available. They are used on a patient only once and then discarded. Needless to say, the chances of infection are greatly reduced, if not eliminated, when disposables are used.

After recommending high colonics for over forty years, I have concluded that a truly competent high colonic therapist is as valuable in the restoration of health as a highly skilled surgeon. Although the procedure is not as admired, and the techniques not as involved, the value of a colonic can, at times, be immeasurable. In some cases, it may even help to avoid surgical intervention. In severe or stubborn psoriatic-eczema conditions, I do not hesitate to recommend this form of hydrotherapy. One of my patients, having been on the regimen for two months without any appreciable results and having failed to respond as quickly as I had expected, took heed of my prodding and had two colonic irrigations in one week. Results were almost immediate. She began to clear up quickly, and within two more months her skin was free of all lesions. It has remained clear ever since. She remarked to me that the turning point was when she had the two colonic irrigations. It was from that moment that she knew she was going to be well. (See the case of M.F. in the photo section.)

The extremes to which opponents of colonic irrigation go to make their point never fail to amaze me. They talk of the possibility of depletion of sodium and dehydration, the possibility of bowel infection, and the possibility of destroying the bacterial flora necessary for normal bowel function. Their biggest argument seems to be that the patient may become dependent on colonics from overuse.

To say that these possibilities do not exist is just as ridiculous. Of course, they exist—as do surgical mishaps and dangerous side effects from drugs—in spite of all necessary precautions being taken. Statistically, there is far less chance of any harm befalling a patient from a colonic than from drugs or surgical procedures. The admitted potential dangers of MTX and PUVA are well known and well documented, yet both are widely used in leading psoriatic centers as well as in private practices. In more than forty years in clinical practice, I have never had a patient who experienced a mishap due to a colonic irrigation; in fact, nothing short of miracles occurred on many occasions.

My patients have only a few colonics over a seven- to eight-week period. Then they follow up with a colonic once every few months until the psoriatic condition clears. As a maintenance measure, another colonic is administered after six months, if necessary. If a patient is totally opposed to a colonic irrigation, however, it is not mandatory. Home enemas can also be very effective. (A colonic should be administered only under the approval of the patient's personal physician.)

High colonics are not advised for children or teenagers under the age of sixteen. In such cases, I recommend gently applied home enemas using a ball syringe with warm water, or a Fleet Enema, available in most pharmacies.

## Home Enemas

If for any reason a patient cannot have a high colonic, I advise a home enema. The difference between a high colonic and a home enema is that an enema usually cleans only the descending and sigmoid segments of the colon (about ten to twelve inches), whereas the high colonic cleans out the transverse and ascending colon as well.

Another obvious difference is that a professional colonic, in most cases, must be performed by an operator at a specific time and at a designated facility, whereas a home enema may be applied in the privacy of one's own home when it is convenient. Last, the expense must be considered, especially if several colonics are required. Colonics can cost anywhere from $50 to $100 each, depending on the facility's location. A home enema, unless it is administered by a professional, is nominal in cost.

I include here a technique developed by one of my former psoriasis patients who suffered from the disease for over twenty years. As a result of applying this method faithfully, her skin condition improved dramatically.

She would lie on her back in an empty bathtub, administer a home enema, and retain the water in her colon for as long as possible before evacuating. While in this position, she would do gentle exercises—knees to chest, elbows to knees, upside-down bicycle, and so forth—and then lie back with her knees up and massage the area of the colon, from side to side. This is a most effective way to stimulate the peristaltic action of the colon as well as to break away any fecal accumulations that may exist on the walls of the colon.

The patient warns, "Be ready to abandon ship at a moment's notice!" but advises that "after a few practice sessions, anyone can do it easily." She administered an enema an average of twice a week.

After practicing this procedure for four months in addition to following the measures in the regimen, she found the massive psoriatic areas on her back greatly improved, with no scars remaining. After this period of time, enemas were no longer required. Photographs taken two years later showed further improvement. (See the case of L.G. in the photo section.)

## The Three-Day Apple Diet

To ensure maximum cleansing of toxins from the system, the Three-Day Apple Diet outlined below should be followed *before* having the colonic or the enema. (I have modified the original Edgar Cayce instructions for the diet.)

### DAY ONE

First thing in the morning: Drink a glass of warm water to which the juice of one fresh lemon has been added.

One hour later, begin the following: Throughout the day, drink plenty of water and eat as many Red or Golden Delicious apples as desired. Most of my patients eat between six and eight apples on the first day of this diet.

Late in the afternoon or in the evening: A high colonic is recommended, if at all possible. If not, a thorough home enema is advised. The purpose of having an enema at this time is to clear out the toxins that have already begun to accumulate in the lower intestinal tract. In the evening, drink one tablespoon of pure olive oil (preferably organic), either plain or mixed into hot water or apple juice.

*Note:* If a full tablespoon of olive oil upsets the stomach, I recommend reducing the amount to one teaspoon. Even this amount may be intolerable if you suffer from either a gallbladder or a liver condition. (Omit the olive oil if adverse reactions occur.)

## DAY TWO
Repeat all of the instructions given for day one, except that a home enema is recommended instead of a high colonic.

## DAY THREE
Repeat all of the instructions given for day one. It is most important that a high colonic or enema be given at the end of day three.

At the completion of this three-day cycle, eat a pint of plain yogurt, which will help to replace the normal bacterial flora of the intestinal tract. An hour later, if hunger persists, begin to follow the dietary suggestions outlined in chapter 6 and appendix A, which allow a greater variety of foods.

### Apples Are Not for Everyone
Without question, some people cannot tolerate apples, raw or cooked, no matter how they are prepared. Apples can cause intestinal discomfort or even severe allergic reactions in some people. If this is the case, the Apple Diet should not even be attempted. There are those, however, who can tolerate apples to a certain degree, but not for three days. Under these circumstances, I recommend going on the diet for one full day instead of three days, and in the evening taking one tablespoon of olive oil. On the next day, I recommend either a home enema or a high colonic.

If, during this cleansing period, you experience weakness, dizziness, or any other adverse reactions, stop the Apple Diet and replace it with the more liberal cleansing diet discussed in chapter 6 and appendix A. Such weakness or dizziness may be the result of a drop in blood sugar. These reactions are often relieved immediately by drinking a glass of orange juice, taking a tablespoon of pure honey, or eating a pint of plain yogurt.

At the end of either the One-Day or the Three-Day Apple Diet, the patient begins to follow the dietary measures set forth in chapter 6 and appendix A.

### Alternatives to the Apple Diet
For those who know they cannot tolerate apples or are allergic to them, there are alternatives: the Grape Diet, the Citrus Diet, or the Fresh Fruit Diet. The steps in these diets are almost identical to those in the Apple Diet.

### THE GRAPE DIET

On this diet, eat as many grapes as desired for three days and drink at least six to eight glasses of pure water daily. Almost any type of grape may be eaten, but I recommend the seedless black Concord variety.

Late in the afternoon or evening on the first and second days of this diet, a thorough home enema is advised. In addition, each evening, one tablespoon of pure olive oil should be taken, either plain or mixed into hot water, grape juice, or any other fruit juice. On the third day, a high colonic should be professionally administered late in the afternoon or evening, if possible. Again, a thorough home enema may be substituted. This is to be followed by consuming a pint of plain yogurt. One hour later, the patient may proceed with the dietary suggestions outlined in chapter 6 and appendix A.

### THE CITRUS DIET

The Citrus Diet consists primarily of tropical and subtropical fruits. The most common of these are oranges, grapefruit, lemons, limes, tangerines, kumquats, mandarins, tangelos, and pomelos. This diet should be followed for five days instead of three. You may eat an unlimited amount of these specific fruits in addition to drinking six to eight glasses of pure water daily.

The ideal procedure would be to have a high colonic administered late in the afternoon or evening of the first and fifth days, and on the third day, a home enema. If high colonics are not available, I suggest having home enemas on the first, third, and fifth days. Each evening, one tablespoon of pure olive oil should be taken, either plain, mixed with hot water, or mixed with any citrus fruit juice.

At the end of the five-day cycle, a pint of plain yogurt should be consumed, and an hour after that, the patient should commence the dietary measures outlined in chapter 6 and appendix A.

*Note:* As with apples, some people are hypersensitive to citrus. If this is the case, avoid the Citrus Diet. All cases of eczema and psoriatic arthritis must avoid citrus fruits and citrus fruit juices.

### THE FRESH FRUIT DIET

The Fresh Fruit Diet is exactly what the name implies. All fruits may be eaten in any quantity on a daily basis, in addition to all the pure water that you can drink. This diet is maintained for a period of either three or five days.

The advantage of choosing this diet over the others is that it is more filling and satisfying and offers greater variety, and the fresh fruits may be eaten raw or cooked. The only restriction as to the choice of fruits, according to the Cayce material, is that all varieties of melons, raw apples, and bananas must be eaten separately rather than mixed with other fruits. Strawberries should not be eaten if there is an underlying condition of arthritis or eczema.

If you choose the three-day Fresh Fruit Diet, a home enema should be applied late in the afternoon or in the evening of the first and second days, and a high colonic should be administered on the third day. If it is not possible to get a colonic, another home enema may be substituted.

If you follow the five-day diet, a high colonic or home enema should be administered on the first and fifth days. A pint of yogurt is to be consumed after the last colonic or enema. An hour later, you can begin a more varied and satisfying diet with the foods designated in chapter 6 and appendix A. During this three- or five-day period, a tablespoon of pure olive oil is taken each evening.

Not only do these diets rid the body of an enormous amount of toxins, but patients also experience a weight loss of five to six pounds or more.

*Note:* If either dizziness or weakness occurs during this cleansing period, or if a person continues to have hunger pangs, I advise adding either a large green leafy salad or a scoop of low-fat cottage cheese, low-fat yogurt, or sugarless Jell-O to the diet. These additional foods help to provide more bulk.

If there is any question as to whether a person can follow any of these cleansing diets, I insist that he or she consult with a medical doctor before commencing. Some may not be able to follow these diets safely if, in addition to psoriasis, they are diabetic, hypoglycemic, have candida, or have diverticulitis.

## The Importance of Water

When one realizes that the body is primarily made up of water, it is not hard to fully recognize how vital this element is to all of the body's chemical processes. This is a biological fact from birth to death. In the embryo, water constitutes 90 percent of the body's weight. In the adult, water makes up 73 percent, discounting fat. As a person gets older, the percentage diminishes even more. In general, it is safe to say that water constitutes anywhere from two-thirds to three-quarters of the human body.

Without this universal medium in which all living biological transactions occur, life is not possible. Among other things, it is the most important cleansing element of the body. The tissues are bathed, the intestines are purified, the body temperature is regulated, and the body humors are maintained. Other functions, too numerous to mention, are dependent on bodily water. Obviously, water intake is of the utmost importance in internal cleansing. Our water intake is derived primarily from food, secondarily from beverages, and lastly from oxidation processes such as fat burning, which produce a lesser amount of water but are nonetheless a major source.

To repeat: The recommended daily intake of water is six to eight glasses, in addition to all other liquids consumed. Water should be drunk before and after meals, which will not only ensure proper digestion, but will also help flush the kidneys, thereby draining accumulations of uric acid.

Needless to say, the purer the water, the better it is. Because of all the various chemical additives in city water today, plus the continued pollution of our natural water sources, I recommend a home water-filtering system or any mountain-spring water that is considered to be pure.

Distilled water may be used in this regimen primarily as the purest form of water, but it should be taken in limited quantities. Of the six to eight glasses of water recommended daily, distilled water should constitute no more than one or two glasses. I am still of the belief that distilled water may drain needed vitamins and minerals from the body.

## Natural Cathartics (Laxatives)

A cathartic is a purgative used to produce an evacuation of the bowel. Some are medicinal, others are natural. It is the latter type that I deal with and, when necessary, strongly advise my patients to use. The colonic or enema cleans out the large intestine or the colon; the natural cathartic cleans out the upper intestinal tract as well. Combined, these two methods are the most effective procedures to cleanse the entire alimentary canal, from stomach to bowel.

Nature's best cathartics are raw fruits and vegetables. Stewed fruits are also quite effective and should be eaten as often as possible. The most beneficial fruits for stewing are figs, apples, raisins, apricots, pears, peaches, and prunes. They may be mixed together, if desired, and a one-half-to one-cup serving should be eaten twice a day until a complete evacuation takes place. Thereafter, making stewed fruits part of one's daily diet will help to keep the system cleansed while supplying the body with natural sugars.

In the case of fruits with a seedy nature—figs, raisins, and so forth—the intestinal movements are mechanically stimulated by the action of the indigestible portion of the fruit residue (seeds). These seeds stimulate local reflexes in the nerves of the intestinal walls. The skins from fresh fruit and the cellulose from raw vegetables, whole wheat, and bran all serve to stimulate the intestines by increasing bulk and, consequently, the degree of stretch of the walls of the bowel.

Foods rich in vitamin B are especially advised, not only because of the nutritional value they provide, but because of the little-known fact that vitamin B aids in cleansing the bowel. From *The Living Body* by Charles Best and Norman Taylor, we learn, "Vitamin B, and other factors of the B Complex, tend to increase the tone of the intestinal musculature, and thus favor natural movements of evacuation."

According to modern nutritionists, foods rich in vitamins B and B complex include wheat germ, brewer's yeast, whole raw barley, soybean flour, whole wheat flour, buckwheat, raw peas, egg yolks, rye bread, almonds, fish, poultry, honey, turnips, beets, dandelions, leafy green vegetables, and broccoli.

## Effective Combinations

Senokot, a natural vegetable laxative derived from the senna leaf, in granular or pill form, is a natural, non-habit-forming cathartic. A teaspoon of Senokot mixed in a glass of warm prune juice is an exceptionally effective laxative. I advise some of my patients to drink this combination at least once a day until they have a complete evacuation. Prune juice is not recommended, however, for those who are diabetic. If this is the case, Senokot should be mixed in a glass of warm water.

Fletcher's Castoria, combined with syrup made from California figs, is another excellent eliminant. One teaspoon of Castoria should be removed from a six-ounce bottle and replaced with one teaspoon of syrup of figs. (From a twelve-ounce bottle, two teaspoons should be removed and replaced with two teaspoons of the syrup.) Before being taken, the bottle is well shaken. My patients then take a half teaspoon of this mixture every half hour until they have a complete evacuation.

Alternating Castoria and syrup of figs by taking them separately is also an effective method. In other words, a patient takes a half teaspoon of Castoria, then one half to one hour later a half teaspoon of syrup of figs. This cycle should be continued until a complete evacuation occurs.

*Note:* Syrup of figs is prepared by soaking five or six California figs in a pot of cold water for a few hours. The water should completely cover the figs by four or five inches. Bring this to a boil, then lower the heat to a simmer. Allow the figs to simmer, covered, for approximately fifty minutes. If too much evaporation takes place after fifteen minutes, add more water. The figs are eaten stewed and the liquid (syrup) is placed in a jar and refrigerated after cooling.

Another effective combination is an orange juice "sandwich." For centuries, castor oil has been a well-known, effective means of purging toxins from the body. For those who find it difficult to take by itself, the way to make it not only effective but also palatable is to combine it with orange juice. Two ounces of orange juice are poured into a six-ounce glass, then the glass is tilted and one ounce of castor oil is slowly added to the orange juice. This is then topped off by slowly adding another two ounces of orange juice. The castor oil will remain suspended between the two layers of orange juice, thus making an orange juice sandwich. Taking castor oil in this manner makes it easier to swallow. Apple juice may be substituted for orange juice, and olive oil or cod liver oil may take the place of castor oil.

Zilatone, Innerclean, and psyllium husks are additional eliminants that are recommended. These products are sometimes available in health food stores and can be purchased through the Cayce product suppliers, listed in appendix D.

Eno Salts, a fruit-based product, is another recommended natural laxative, as is milk of magnesia, both of which are alkaline in nature.

There are many other safe, non-habit-forming eliminants on the market today. For the best results, it is advisable to alternate them by using a vegetable-based eliminant on one day and a fruit-based eliminant on another day.

## Olive Oil

Olive oil, taken by itself, is a very practical and effective cathartic. I advise my patients to take a half-teaspoon of olive oil approximately three or four times a day until it produces a good bowel movement. If you have a gallbladder condition, smaller doses are suggested.

Olive oil, taken internally, has recently been recognized by the scientific community as being effective in preventing cholesterol buildup on the arterial walls. This oil has also been credited with supplying nutrients to the digestive tract, aiding in elimination, and acting as an intestinal food.

As a gentle enema, olive oil is also recommended for a thorough cleansing of the colon. To relax the colon, applying a home enema using a half-pint of pure olive oil with no other additives is often effective. After a complete evacuation occurs, a follow-up enema using warm water is suggested. As a final rinse, one tablespoon of Glyco-Thymoline (an alkaline cleansing mouthwash) should be added to a quart and a half of body-temperature water. This final cleansing measure will prevent a generalized "weakening" state. I recommend this procedure be carried out by my patients once or twice a week, especially in cases of chronic constipation or stubborn psoriasis.

## The Tri-Salts

This mixture has been advised in the Cayce readings as another effective cleansing agent for psoriasis sufferers. It is made up of equal parts sulfur, cream of tartar, and Rochelle salts. This product is sold as Sulflax and is available from the Heritage Store and from Baar Products (see appendix D). People who decide to use it are advised to take one teaspoon every morning as directed on the label. Although Sulflax is a nonprescription item, it should be administered under the direction of an osteopath or a medical doctor.

## High-Fiber Foods

The importance of high-fiber foods in today's diet cannot be overemphasized. These foods are highly advisable, for they help to stimulate peristaltic action throughout the intestinal tract and cleanse the colon by virtue of their coarse action on the walls.

Recent years have brought about increased awareness of the value of high-fiber foods in the prevention of colon cancer. The *New England Journal of Medicine* published a report stating that researchers at the University of Modena in Italy believe high-fiber foods possibly prevent colon cancer, as well as heart disease, by lowering blood levels of cholesterol. The researchers believe that one reason for this is that high-fiber diets speed up the movement of food through the small intestine, thereby preventing certain disease processes from taking hold. The Associated Press released an article in June 1982 reporting findings by a panel of scientists, based on a two-year study for the National Academy of Sciences, indicating that a diet high in fiber supplied by whole-grain cereals, fruits, and vegetables may inhibit certain cancers.

Although these scientists claim that their findings are inconclusive, the fact remains that fiber-rich foods have a cleansing effect throughout the colon because of their inability to be digested. Fibrous-type foods (roughage) speed up the process of waste elimination, and the destructive, possibly even cancerous, elements do not have time to gain a foothold in the large intestine before they are scraped off the walls of the colon and passed out of the body. These conclusions parallel those of the researchers from the University of Modena.

The most common high-fiber foods are whole- or cracked-wheat breads, whole-grain breakfast cereals, fresh fruits and vegetables, and almonds. The almond is of particular benefit because it is high in fiber and alkaline in nature. Almonds may be eaten raw (preferably two to four each day for at least three days a week), in baked goods, or in other food preparations.

It is most important that fiber-rich foods be included, whenever possible, in the daily diet. These food items help reduce the transit time of fecal material in the bowel, helping the toxic elements (waste) to be excreted in the normal twenty-four to thirty-six hours. If the transit time of impurities is allowed to go beyond thirty-six hours before exiting the body, backup pressure occurs, which can lead to irritability of the intestinal tract, which, in turn, may lead to anything from an annoyance to a life-threatening illness.

Examples of fiber-rich breakfast foods include Miller's Bran, All-Bran, oat bran, Wheat Chex, Wheaties, Grape-Nuts, and unsweetened shredded wheat. Some fiber-rich vegetables are green beans, cauliflower, carrots, lettuce, sweet potatoes, celery, and cabbage (green and red). Other foods that help gastrointestinal function and detoxification are pectin (in apples), agar, psyllium, guar, malt extract, and olive oil. Of these, psyllium husk fiber is considered to be the most beneficial. (*Note:* Fiber-rich foods bind water; therefore, adequate liquid intake is essential.)

## Fume and Steam Baths

One of the oldest forms of body rejuvenation, cleansing, and stimulation of the skin is the ancient fume or steam bath. The purpose behind taking this form of hydrotherapy (if available) is to open the pores in order to aid in the removal of toxins through the sweat glands of the skin. If the skin is extremely sensitive and almost tissue-thin, as often occurs in severe exfoliative psoriasis, I do not recommend steam. Fortunately, these very extreme cases are rare. This type of hydrotherapy can be undertaken either by purchasing a home unit or by using those found at spas and health clubs. A word of caution: If a person suffers from a heart problem, high blood pressure, or from any other questionable systemic condition, using a steam room or a steam cabinet is *not* advised.

Even if there is no reason to expect an adverse reaction to steam, I still advise that an attendant be on hand to apply cool towels to the head and neck, in case the person becomes overheated while in the steam cabinet. The cabinet encloses the whole body but leaves the head exposed to permit sufficient oxygen intake. A person sits in this specially made unit while steam is generated and engulfs the entire body.

For psoriatic conditions, Cayce advised that a mixture of one tablespoon of witch hazel and half a pint of water be placed in the reservoir of the steam cabinet. The average time limit for remaining in a steam cabinet is twenty to thirty minutes. This may vary five minutes either way. It is important to learn how much steam a patient can tolerate without any adverse effects. It is best to shower with plain warm water after having a steam or fume bath. Avoid using soap, which tends to clog the pores of the skin again.

A large amount of body fluid is lost during a steam or fume bath. Each person has a different tolerance and reaction to this loss of fluid. If the loss becomes excessive, the reaction is similar to that of a person suffering from heat prostration, and the same treatment is called for. The classic signs are fainting, dizziness, and weakness. It is vital to replace the salt lost from the tissue cells. Therefore, make sure the person drinks a glass of water to which a pinch of salt has been added, both before and after having a steam bath, as well as one or two glasses of pure water while taking the steam. To prevent any loss of potassium and calcium, it is best to eat foods rich in these minerals both before and after this form of therapy.

I can't help but recall the adverse reaction one of my former patients experienced from loss of salt. After traveling on an extremely hot day in a non-air-conditioned bus and feeling totally exhausted, she went for a scheduled steam bath. While in the steam cabinet, she felt faint and weak. The attendant in charge immediately removed her from the cabinet and called to inform me of her reaction. I suggested that he give her a glass of water to which a quarter teaspoon of salt had been added. Upon drinking the water, she found that her faintness and weakness disappeared almost instantaneously. This is akin to the experience of athletes who take salt tablets on hot days to replace any salt they might lose through profuse sweating.

## Saffron Tea or Saffron Water and Steam Baths

Another measure I suggest that will help patients derive the greatest benefit from steam is to drink a cup of saffron tea or a six- to eight-ounce glass of saffron water about thirty minutes to an hour before taking the steam bath. The steam will open the pores of the skin, and the saffron tea or water will work its way right through the skin, carrying toxins along with it, thus aiding in the internal cleansing process. I consider this a most valuable procedure to follow if you have access to a steam bath. Both saffron tea and saffron water are covered in chapter 7.

The precautions are basically the same as for Epsom salts baths. No cardiovascular case should have a steam or fume bath, and there should always be an attendant on hand to watch the reaction and be prepared to administer assistance, if necessary. If the skin is too sensitive with the addition of witch hazel, plain steam may be all that can be used in the beginning. I do not recommend sauna baths be taken in cases of psoriasis or eczema, unless it is a wet sauna.

Each person must judge what can or cannot be tolerated. I advise all who inquire to check with their own doctors before attempting the fume or steam bath. Effective as these therapies are, they may be harmful to some.

## Exercise

Exercise is a vital part of the regimen for clearing psoriasis. It stimulates the internal structures of the body, increases circulation, activates the glands, oxygenates the blood, opens the pores, pumps the lymph, and filters the blood through the liver and the kidneys.

Exercising, especially in the open air, provides untold benefits. I encourage my patients to participate in noncontact sports such as tennis, badminton, golf, jogging (moderately), walking, and swimming. Contact sports should be avoided because psoriatics have a sensitive dermal layer of the skin. You may recall it is often noted that the disease first appears after there is a bruise to the skin.

Bicycling, either outdoors or on a stationary home unit, rowing, and low-impact aerobics, at home or in a health club, are additional forms of exercise that are beneficial to the psoriatic and should be done on a regular basis, two or three times a week. Stretching exercises also aid the body in eliminating waste matter more effectively, but for those who have psoriasis, it must be remembered that stretching may also traumatize the sensitive layers of the skin; therefore, this should be done gently and in moderation. Social dancing stimulates all internal structures, and consequently, also helps in the cleansing process.

The most effective type of walking is brisk walking, outdoors, rain or shine. Rhythmic breathing while walking doubles its effectiveness. This is accomplished by inhaling for six counts, holding your breath for six counts, and then exhaling for six counts. Doing this will help you to develop a pattern in your daily walking routine. If possible, set a specific time for walking each day and never walk to the point of exhaustion. When you walk, the mind should be free of any nagging problems, or the desired benefits will be lost in the murk and mire of destructive thinking.

It has been suggested that if you want to prevent a heart attack, you should get yourself a dog. Why? Because you will have to regularly walk your dog. Many of us neglect to do any walking, especially in the evening, because we prefer to watch television. Having a dog forces us out of this sedentary habit.

I can personally vouch for this advice, for there have been many instances when, after a full day of seeing patients, the last thing I wanted to do was walk my dog, Shane. But he would look up at me with soulful eyes as if to say, "Okay, now it's time to take care of me." I would drag myself out of my chair to get his leash, stagger through the door, and begin our walk. Before long, a new consciousness of well-being would come over me. Where did the tiredness disappear to, and where did my renewed energy come from? Perhaps it came from the production of endorphins, a benefit discovered by the jogging set. Whatever the reason, once I started walking, I felt different, oxygenated, and alert. I realized suddenly that I had not been taking care of Shane—he was taking care of me!

Swimming has long been recognized as a most beneficial sport and physical activity, provided that the water you swim in is free of pollution. It is so effective because it works every muscle, joint, and ligament of the body. It also aids respiration, circulation, and flexibility, which is one of the most important elements in warding off old age and its associated stiffness. Swimming in clear water, especially clean ocean water, cleanses and stimulates the skin, thereby helping to wash away toxins. The benefits are too numerous to mention. Make swimming a part of your life, and vigor and vitality will accompany you wherever you go. An aura of youthfulness will surround you—and if you radiate health, health will most surely accompany you all the days of your life.

Find time to exercise, or nature will eventually provide you with nothing but time—flat on your back!

## Detox

The purpose of the aforementioned diets, cathartics, and cleansing methods can be expressed in one word: *detoxification*. These cover only some of the available options that I have presented to my patients.

Some options are more effective than others for different individuals. Determining the most effective ones is best done by the attending physician and the patient.

My experience in dealing with psoriasis for so many years leads me to the undeniable conclusion that psoriasis is a backup system in action. It is your skin struggling to do the job of another organ. Keep in mind, psoriasis is not burned off or rubbed off; it is flushed out!.

# CHAPTER 6

# Diet and Nutrition Basics

D octor, does my diet have anything to do with my condition?"
is a question most often asked by the average person suffering
from psoriasis. In practically every case, the answer most frequently
given by orthodox physicians is "No, diet has nothing to do with it."
So the patient goes on eating whatever he or she wants, gets worse and
worse, and is prescribed drug after drug. This attitude is limited not
only to the United States, but it is prevalent throughout the world.
I can attest to that, having lectured on the subject on five continents
with the same sad story coming in from members of my audience.
How tragic, how unnecessary, whereas, more often than not, with
changes to a healthy diet, the sufferer can change the tide and live a
life free of the burden of psoriasis.

In this chapter, the answers to the role diet plays in psoriasis, as
I have witnessed, is clearly outlined. It is up to the patients to follow
through or to ignore. Their decision will determine their future.

## My Introduction to Psoriasis

I met Mr. H. while interning in Denver, Colorado. Before then, my
knowledge of psoriasis had been limited to textbook photographs and
descriptions. Here, for the first time, I saw psoriasis "in the flesh."

"Covered from head to toe" is the only way to describe Mr. H.'s
condition. Throughout his life, he had been unsuccessfully searching

for help. His desperate plea aroused my interest to the point where I began gathering all available information I could on this disease. It marked the beginning of my research into one of mankind's most disfiguring skin problems.

We were not successful in treating Mr. H. at that time. The only, temporary, benefit he received was derived from the sun-filled days of Colorado. He left the hospital knowing full well that the lesions would soon return, as they had done in the past.

Fifteen years elapsed before I contacted Mr. H. again, for, by then, I had successfully treated several psoriasis cases. While our reunion was joyous, I was shocked by his appearance. He was a mere shadow of his former self, looking gaunt and tired and decidedly underweight. The spring was gone from his step. His every movement was slow and deliberate, and his speech was that of a man who had been through the mill. Five years earlier, he had suffered a massive heart attack and was hospitalized for several weeks with little hope of recovery. Miraculously, however, he pulled through, but only to lead a life bordering on invalidism.

Mr. H. was still suffering from psoriasis. Upon examining him, I found his lesions to be just as extensive and severe as ever. I showed him before-and-after photographs of my patients, and he expressed particular interest when I explained the significant role played by diet in alleviating psoriasis, something of which we had been unaware fifteen years earlier. The story he then told me lent credence to the entire theory.

During his hospital stay, he was fed intravenously for several weeks. During this period, a miracle seemed to take place: his psoriasis completely disappeared. The doctors had no explanation, and he was equally amazed. Not even a trace of the lesions remained, and since no one knew the reason for this unusual occurrence, it was simply considered extraordinary and forgotten. Mr. H. related that upon being discharged from the hospital, he was still perfectly clear of any lesions and went home to his usual diet. In no time at all, the psoriasis returned with a vengeance.

"What is your normal diet?" I asked. "Rare roast beef and tomatoes," he replied. "I eat tomatoes by the bushel!" Unfortunately, it will never be known whether Mr. H. could have benefited from my regimen, for he died shortly after my visit of an apparent second heart attack.

The fact is that for the relatively short period of time Mr. H. was fed intravenously, he did not eat two of the major restricted items of my regimen's diet, red meat and tomatoes. This allowed his body time to detoxify. As a result, the lesions disappeared.

I contend that in severe cases of psoriasis, a medically supervised period of intravenous feeding could accelerate the detoxification process. This, however, is for medical authorities to decide. In my opinion, an experience such as that of Mr. H., as well as those reported by other patients, seems to justify further empirical studies. Someday, techniques such as intravenous feeding for detoxifying the body may be looked upon as a primary therapy for many diseases.

## Rules of the Road

In the management and control of psoriasis, the significance of an effective diet has been questioned for as long as the disease has been researched. The fact is, as early as 1932, the effect of diet on psoriasis was clearly demonstrated by Jay F. Schamberg, MD, a former professor of dermatology at the University of Pennsylvania. His work, however, was largely overlooked and seems to have faded into oblivion.

This controversial issue of diet has caused much confusion and bewilderment. Since authorities constantly contradict one another, people are often left in a dietary dilemma. In most cases, they would be eager to follow a nutritional program if one were available to them. Should a physician mention diet, it is usually only in a cursory manner, or merely to dismiss it as having little or no effect in alleviating this disease. I believe the scientific community needs to become more cognizant of the intrinsic value of diet. My research and treatment have proven to me, beyond question, that diet not only plays a distinct role but is, indeed, the most important factor in healing psoriasis. Besides being the very foundation of the recommended therapy, it is also the key factor in preventing its recurrence.

In all the years that I have been treating psoriasis cases, I have never achieved a successful result if my regimen's diet was not followed to at least a reasonable degree. Other recommended measures are valuable and certainly assist in hastening positive results in healing this skin disorder. Without the underlying common denominator of proper diet, however, the effort is fruitless. If this statement sounds like an exaggerated claim, I can assure you it is not. A psoriatic must fully accept and understand that the consumption or avoidance of certain foods is vital to his recovery from this dermatological problem. If a patient is unwilling to accept this fact, it may be necessary to revert back to the more orthodox forms of therapy rather than the alternative route presented here.

I do not wish to mislead my readers into believing that the recommended measures, including the suggested diet, guarantee success. There are a variety of reasons for failure. In many cases, however, those who did not receive beneficial results were people who refused to alter their dietary habits, or if they did follow the prescribed diet, did not do so for a long enough period of time. When I begin to sense this attitude in patients, usually after a few visits, I discourage them from continuing. My efforts are reserved for those who are at least willing to give this more natural approach time and an opportunity to work. Those who say that they will try to go on the diet for a few weeks are rarely successful. Most seem to forget that it took considerable time to pollute every cell of their body's tissue before the poisons bulged through their skin in the form of psoriasis. Yet, once the cleansing process takes effect, it is amazing how often the body responds quickly, in a matter of months, sometimes weeks. The most devastating lesions simply seem to dry up and disappear once the body is given the proper tools with which to work.

Granted, there are some who developed psoriatic lesions and experienced a complete remission of the disease for unknown reasons. There are also those who simply rubbed salves or ointments on their skin and achieved similar results. Needless to say, these cases do not have to be concerned with extensive therapies or diets. It would be well for them to remember, however, that they are prone to the disease, if only to a minor degree, and should therefore cultivate and develop an awareness of which foods are beneficial to them, as well as those that are detrimental.

The psoriatics with whom I am most concerned are those who are chronically plagued with the disease; those who have sought relief for many years—some for most of their lives. They reach an impenetrable barrier when seeking explanations as to its cause and a therapy that is relatively risk-free, successful, and lasting. I reach out to these sufferers and passionately declare that there are answers to their problem, in both cause and management, the most important of which is found in their daily diet.

When Cayce was asked if there was an absolute cure for psoriasis, his answer was straight and to the point: most of this is found in diet. There is a cure. It requires patience, persistence, and right thinking.

The idea of an illness such as psoriasis responding favorably to changes in diet no longer seems remote or bizarre. Has it not been said for ages that we are what we eat? This holds true, particularly in the case of psoriatics. Fortunately, as human beings, to a large extent we have the power to control both what we think and what we eat.

At this point I wish to interject what I feel is an important awareness for patients as well as the general public: whenever possible, always choose certified organic foods, whether they are meats, fruits, vegetable, or dairy products. They are foods that are grown or raised without the use of pesticides, preservatives, hormones, or other artificial substances that are consequently absorbed by the consumer.

## The Acid-Alkaline Balance

What is it about diet that is so vital to the psoriatic? It is the importance of maintaining the proper acid-alkaline (base) balance of the body's chemistry. Although this subject was briefly touched on in an earlier chapter, it is of such value that it warrants discussing in more detail.

For the preservation of good health, nature demands that the body remain more on the alkaline side than the acid side. The body becomes more resistant to all types of disease and physical ailments when engulfed in an internal chemical atmosphere that is alkaline. Arthritic joints are greatly relieved, colds and congestion are counteracted, skin problems diminish, and internal organs become less burdened.

It must not be assumed that acids are not important, for they most certainly are, but in their proper proportion.

## The 80/20 Percent Food Ratio

A person's blood should always be slightly alkaline, with a pH of 7.3 to 7.5 in chemical reaction, to maintain the optimum in general health and immunity. This is primarily maintained by the body's natural lines of defense and is influenced by the foods ingested as well as one's emotional makeup. In later chapters we will explore the effects generated by destructive thoughts and negative emotions. Food intake and the tremendous influence this has on the psoriatic are what shall concern us in this section.

The psoriatic, psoriatic arthritic, and/or eczematous patient should keep before his or her mind's eye the ratio of 80/20 percent at all times. This means that the daily diet should consist of 80 percent alkaline-forming foods and 20 percent acid-forming foods, or, to state it more simply, many more alkaline- than acid-forming foods should be consumed.

For most of us, our eating habits are just the opposite. We fill ourselves with acid-forming foods, which produce a hyperacidic condition, and then wonder why our joints are stiff in the morning, we are more susceptible to colds, and we develop skin blemishes, especially as we get older. This is because the acids become overabundant in the body and the cells cry out for relief. It is amazing to see how quickly a patient responds, in a positive way, when the shift from acidity to alkalinity takes place. Joints become more flexible and less painful, colds and congestion as well as some allergies often clear up, and the skin takes on a healthier glow, with many blemishes disappearing. Results are lasting if a patient does not revert back to his or her previous eating habits after being relieved of these conditions.

It is obviously mandatory to learn which foods are alkaline and which are acid, as well as which should be avoided altogether, such as the nightshades and most saturated fats and sweets.

There have been occasions when, unknowingly, some of my patients gradually lost track of maintaining the 80–20 percent ratio of foods. They found themselves eating more of the 20 percent of acid formers than they should, simply because they were listed as "allowed" foods. Lesions gradually began to resurface without the patients' realizing why. Once their diet was altered to include more alkaline formers than acid formers, the lesions slowly began to subside.

Additionally, specific habits and physical activities have an influence on acid-alkaline reactions in the body. Recognizing whether those habits are beneficial or harmful is of the utmost importance. This subject will be covered in more detail as we proceed.

# Alkaline Formers versus Acid Formers

Modern nutritionists agree that, in general, fruits are the primary *cleansers* of the body, while vegetables are considered to be the *builders*.

*All* foods are either alkaline forming, acid forming, or neutral. The alkaline formers are the lighter, watery-type foods that are more easily digested, such as fruits and vegetables. The acid formers are the heavier, protein foods, such as meats and grains, which require greater breakdown for proper digestion and absorption. The neutrals are the dairy products, such as milk, yogurt, and kefir. If anything, this group tends toward the alkaline side of the scale.

## Alkaline Formers

Alkaline-forming foods (80 percent of the daily diet) are, as mentioned, the more "watery" types of fruits and vegetables and their juices. Because these foods are broken down more easily by the body, they are more readily digested.

Most fruits are alkaline-forming (reacting) within the body, with the exception of five (cranberries, currants, large prunes, plums, and blueberries) that are acid forming. The benefits and nutrition derived from fresh fruits in general far outweigh the minor acidic content of these few exceptions. I therefore usually advise my patients to eat fresh fruits often, without being overly concerned about their acid-alkaline content, as long as it is not overdone or they do not cause an adverse reaction. Consuming too much fruit or fruit juice can induce elevated triglycerides, because excess fruit sugars can be retained in the body tissues as stored fat. Patients affected with eczema should particularly take this seriously.

In nutritional terms, fruits are divided into three categories: acid, subacid, and sweet. The reader, however, should not be confused by these terms and regard such fruits as acid forming, for, in fact, most so-called acid fruits are actually alkaline reacting in the body.

### Fruits That Should Be Accorded Special Attention

- *Strawberries, citrus fruits,* and *citrus juices* should be avoided in cases of psoriatic arthritis and eczema, or if there is a hypersensitive reaction.

- *Avocados* should be avoided if a patient has gout.

- *Raw apples, melons,* and *bananas* should not be combined with other foods; for example, in fruit salads or on cereals or as part of a regular meal, such as an appetizer or a dessert. These fruits, however, may be eaten separately as a snack or between meals. In other words, eat them alone or leave them alone.

- *Citrus fruits*—oranges, grapefruit, lemons, limes, kumquats, tangerines, and mandarins, and their juices—*should not be combined* with whole grains, dairy products (milk, butter, yogurt, cheese, and so forth), eggs, or white-flour products (such as cereals, breads, muffins, and pancakes). The only exception to this is for particularly active children and for other individuals whose daily activities require them to expend a great deal of energy. These people may combine citrus fruits and juices with whole-grain products (no white-flour products), provided there are no adverse reactions. If the skin becomes hypersensitive or irritated from eating too many citrus fruits, I recommend eliminating them or consuming less of them in favor of noncitrus fruits.

Most vegetables are also alkaline forming (reacting) within the body, except for the following, which are acid forming: mature corn (large kernels), dried corn, rhubarb, winter squash (hubbard, acorn, butternut), and Brussels sprouts. (Legumes such as dried beans and peas; kidney, pinto, black, and navy beans; black-eyed, split, and chickpeas; and lentils are also acid forming.) Although these vegetables are acid reacting, they may still be consumed but in smaller quantities. It is advisable to eat three vegetables that grow above the ground—lettuce, celery, spinach, broccoli, and so forth—to one that grows below the ground—carrots, beets, sweet potatoes, onions, and so forth. (A more detailed chart of above- and below-ground vegetables may be found in appendix A.) It should be noted that consuming an overabundance of any one vegetable, fruit, or juice that is high in vitamins that are stored naturally in the body (vitamins A, D, E, and K) may trigger an adverse reaction. Therefore, moderation should be exercised.

More vitamins and minerals are assimilated by drinking freshly made vegetable juice to which one packet of unflavored gelatin has been added. To obtain the maximum benefit, this juice should be consumed within ten minutes after being prepared.

Beware the nightshades! It is crucial that all psoriatic and eczematous patients familiarize themselves with the term *nightshade*. This represents a family of plants that they should totally avoid regardless of their acid-alkaline reaction. The nightshades are as follows: tomatoes, tobacco, eggplant, white potatoes, peppers, and paprika. This subject will be covered later in this chapter. Suffice it here to simply list them for the sake of recognition.

The following tips also help to increase alkalinity in the body and should, therefore, be incorporated into one's diet and lifestyle:

## Alkaline Formers

- Granular lecithin, an alkaline food supplement, added to foods and beverages. (Lecithin will be covered in more detail later in this chapter.)
- Freshly squeezed lemon juice in a cup of hot or cold water. (Many patients have found this to be a good substitute for hot tea or coffee. Not only does it help maintain the alkalinity, it aids the internal cleansing process.)
- Nutritious fruit juices such as grape, pear, papaya, apricot, guava, mango, and pineapple.
- Grapefruit or orange juice (4 parts) combined with fresh lemon or lime juice (1 part).
- Fresh or stewed fruits.
- Vegetable juices extracted from raw carrots, celery, beets, parsley, romaine lettuce, and spinach (raw onions are particularly cleansing).
- Exercising and physical activities, especially outdoors.
- A bowel movement at least once a day.
- Positive emotions such as self-confidence, kindness, humor, laughter, forgiveness, and so forth.
- Three to five drops of Glyco-Thymoline in a glass of pure water, before bed time, five days per week. (This alkaline cleansing solution will be covered further in this chapter.)
- Cereals. Amaranth, millet, and quinoa are the only alkaline cereals; all others are acidic.

## Acid Formers

Acid-forming foods (20 percent of the daily diet) are the heavier, more solid foods (proteins, starches, sugars, fats, and oils). Combinations of these foods, especially when consumed in large quantities, build up the acid content of the blood and consequently aggravate a psoriatic condition. Meats, grains, cheese, sugars, potatoes, dried peas, beans, oils, butter, cream, and processed meats (frankfurters, salami, bologna, and so forth) are the most common acid formers. These foods require the digestive organs to produce more acids to break them down for absorption.

Depending on the type of food consumed, the body is left with either an *acid ash* or an *alkaline ash*. The ideal chemical reaction is one that tends toward an *alkaline ash,* thus the reasoning behind the 80 percent alkaline/20 percent acid food intake. When acid-forming foods are digested, what remains is called an acid ash. Acid-forming foods, although a relatively small percentage of the recommended daily diet, are nevertheless vital to the body's growth, repair, and development.

The following foods and habits also tend to increase acidity in the body and should, therefore, be avoided as much as possible:

- Too many acid-forming foods at the same meal (for example, starches with sweets, proteins and meats, meats or fats with sugars, too many starchy foods; a list of proteins and starches may be found in appendix A)
- Cane sugar and any product made from cane sugar
- Most types of vinegar, especially wine vinegar and white (grain) vinegar. (The only types permitted is apple cider vinegar.)
- Foods that contain large amounts of preservatives, artificial flavorings, colorings, and additives
- Alcoholic beverages
- Smoking
- Drug abuse
- Constipation
- Inactivity—mental and/or physical
- Negative emotions such as feelings of insecurity, fearfulness, worry, anxiety, jealousy, bitterness, resentment, inferiority, and destructive thoughts in general

# The Effect Toxemia Has on the Acid-Alkaline (Base) Balance

I ask my readers to carefully ponder the following scientific fact revealed in Francis M. Pottenger's *Symptoms of Visceral Disease.* It clearly defines the effect that toxemia (poisons in the blood) has on the acid-alkaline chemistry of the body's tissues: "When toxemia is prolonged, a loss of body bases occurs, which results in a shifting of the acid-alkali balance of the tissues toward the acid side. This has an important bearing on the production and prolongation of toxic symptoms. This condition calls for the administration of alkalis, either in the form of alkaline foods or alkaline salts. This is more marked in some diseases than in others."

Psoriasis is one of those diseases in which there is a decided shift in the body chemistry to the acid side. A psoriasis patient, therefore, must be aware of the significance of maintaining a proper balance and must be willing to follow the suggested diet and regimen for as long as necessary.

## Glyco-Thymoline

Glyco-Thymoline, mentioned in chapter 5, is an intestinal antiseptic and is alkaline. This substance, when taken internally (four or five drops in a glass of water before bedtime, five days per week), is beneficial to the psoriatic, psoriatic arthritic, and eczema sufferer in that it promotes alkalinity and cleanses the digestive tract, which, in turn, reduces toxemia.

In some cases, Glyco-Thymoline, when externally applied full strength to small affected areas, has proven to be quite soothing in relieving severe itching (pruritis).

Although this is a nonprescription item (a mouthwash), when taken internally, it must first be approved by an MD or an osteopath. If this product is unavailable in a local drugstore, readers may order it from Baar Products or the Heritage Store (see appendix D).

## Lecithin

I suggest that all of my psoriasis patients take lecithin regularly. Derived primarily from soybeans, lecithin, rich in nonanimal proteins and highly alkaline, has been considered by many nutritionists to be a fat emulsifier. In simple terms, it prevents blood fat (cholesterol) from accumulating in the arteries by keeping it in suspension. Arteriosclerosis develops from accumulations of fat deposits on the arterial walls. It is believed that lecithin helps to prevent this from happening. Contrary to this concept, however, the value of lecithin is held in dispute, according to an article that appeared in the October 1989 Tufts University newsletter. Tufts University's report states that studies conducted since 1943 indicate that lecithin has no effect in reducing blood cholesterol levels and that claims of its beneficial aspects have no basis in fact.

Other studies, however, do recognize lecithin as a beneficial health measure, including the influence it has on thought processes. German scientists state, "No phosphoric acid—no brain." Phosphorus, in the form of phosphoric acid, is found in lecithin and is essential in human physiology, especially in brain and nerve tissue. Lecithin has been used in therapeutic doses for patients suffering from degenerative diseases such as scleroderma and rheumatoid arthritis, as well as diseases with neurological involvement, such as multiple sclerosis (MS) and amyotrophic lateral sclerosis (ALS).

## Lecithin and Psoriasis

In her book *Let's Get Well,* Adelle Davis referred to psoriasis as an "eczema-like skin condition which appears to result from faulty utilization of fats." This world-renowned nutritionist reported that when 254 psoriasis patients were given four to eight tablespoons of lecithin daily, no new eruptions occurred after the first week, and the most severe cases recovered within five months. She also stated that people with this abnormality usually had excessive amounts of cholesterol in their skin and blood. By the time their blood cholesterol was reduced to normal, their psoriasis was no longer evident. Even though Davis reported these findings, I have personally found with my patients that those with severe psoriasis, more often than not, had perfectly normal blood pictures and, in some cases, a surprisingly low cholesterol count. I make this comparison only to show that the blood picture is not necessarily a key factor in evaluating psoriasis. A blood test known as an SMA-12 or an SMA-24, along with a urinalysis, may show other abnormalities of which a physician should be aware.

In addition to lecithin's being harmless, non–habit forming, alkaline, and an aid in digestion, there is another important benefit, especially to the psoriatic: it has a decided effect on bowel evacuation. I have found that lecithin acts as an excellent natural laxative.

I recommend my adult patients take one tablespoon of granular lecithin three times a day, five days a week. Children are permitted one teaspoon daily unless they are allergic to soy or soy products. It makes no difference how it is consumed: it may be added to water or juice or sprinkled over a salad or cereal. Once a patient's skin is clear, I recommend that the lecithin intake be reduced to one tablespoon a day, five days a week.

Lecithin is readily available in any well-supplied health food store, drugstore, or supermarket and comes in three forms: liquid, tablet, and granular. I prefer granules, because the phosphatide content is highest in this form. It is the phosphatide content of lecithin that emulsifies the blood fat. Admittedly, the liquid capsule form is more convenient and easier to swallow. However, it takes nine capsules (1,200 mg each) to equal the amount of phosphatides found in one level tablespoon of lecithin granules. It should be noted, however, that like all over-the-counter substances, lecithin should not be abused by overuse, for then it may interfere with calcium absorption.

## A Case in Point

As I stated previously, the therapeutic effects of lecithin are far-reaching and sometimes quite surprising. Once, at a dinner party, I sat next to a dear friend and noticed how unusually picky she was regarding the foods that were served. In the past, I had never noticed her being so choosy about the foods she ate, for she always seemed able to enjoy anything and everything. When I inquired why she was particularly selective about her foods, she related that in the past few months she was unable to eat foods that contained fat, particularly milk and animal fats. The reactions of eating these foods produced devastating discomfort in the form of welts, throat constriction, and skin eruptions. There seemed to be no logical explanation for this sudden change in food reactions. I suggested that she consider taking lecithin daily. Even though she was not familiar with this product, she agreed to try it, since it was a natural substance.

When I next met her at a dinner party, she was able to eat anything that was placed before her, with no adverse reactions. She informed me that after beginning to take lecithin, her difficulty with digesting fats stopped almost immediately. Since then, she continues to take lecithin regularly, remains free of the problem, and attributes her recovery entirely to it. It must not be assumed that everyone will have the same reaction from taking lecithin. In this particular case, however, the results were dramatic enough to warrant comment.

## Atmospheric Influence on the Acid-Alkaline Balance

It is common knowledge that most psoriatic conditions usually improve during the summer and get worse in the winter. During the colder months, home-heating units reduce the humidity in the air and subsequently dry out the skin. A humidifier usually corrects this situation. In the summer, because less clothing is worn, beneficial sun rays are allowed to penetrate the skin, which brings about a healing influence. In addition, much more water is normally consumed during the summer months, which aids the internal cleansing process.

It was fascinating for me to come across a series of charts by Dr. S. W. Tromp of the William Peterson Foundation that related physiological processes in the body with observed seasonal changes. In his book *How Atmospheric Conditions Affect Your Health,* author Michel Gauguelin, a science writer and French researcher in psychology and statistics at the Sorbonne, presents these charts, which show the effects that seasons have on the acid-alkaline contents of the gastrointestinal tract. Among the myriad functions listed was the fact that gastroacidity increases in the winter and is low in the summer, whereas gastroalkalinity is high in the summer and low in the winter. This adds credence to the link between acid-alkaline balance and psoriasis.

## Avoiding the Nightshades

As mentioned earlier in this chapter, a psoriatic must become well acquainted with the term *nightshade,* for it denotes a group of the most undesirable substances that should be avoided. Nightshade, as some of my readers may know, is a deadly poison (*Atropa belladonna*).

Most people recognize this simply as belladonna, which is used only for medicinal purposes.

Unprecedented research has been conducted by Norman F. Childers, PhD, formerly of the agricultural department of Rutgers University, who is presently continuing his work at the University of Florida, Institute of Food and Agricultural Sciences at Gainesville, Florida. He has compiled overwhelming evidence that plants of the nightshade family have a most deleterious effect on people afflicted with arthritis and may even be a basic cause. Psoriasis and arthritis, in my opinion, are closely allied diseases, because I have found quite often that they both respond favorably to the regimen contained herein. This is covered in more detail in chapter 16.

### The Nightshades
- Tomatoes (and their derivatives)
- Tobacco
- Eggplant
- White potatoes
- Peppers (except the spice, black pepper)
- Paprika

*Tomatoes.* During my years of research, I have personally observed that many of my psoriatic patients love tomatoes. Before becoming aware of Dr. Childers's findings, I noticed how detrimental tomatoes were to my patients and consequently eliminated them from their diet. As soon as I did, there was a slow but marked improvement in their condition. While corresponding with Dr. Childers, I learned that he, too, achieved similar results. Therefore, tomatoes and their derivatives (juice, ketchup, sauces, and so forth) rank highest in foods to avoid.

*Tobacco.* Since tobacco is also a nightshade plant, smoking should be completely avoided, or at least greatly curtailed. Smoking poisons the respiratory system; contracts small blood vessels, which can lead to heart disease; and, among other factors, has an acidic effect on the body. Those who insist on smoking should try to limit themselves to only a few cigarettes per day.

A recent statistic states that about 25 percent of all psoriasis cases have their origin in smoking. In case you are wondering, secondary smoke is just as harmful as actually smoking yourself.

*White potatoes.* "White" indicates the inside color of the potato. Both the pulp and the skin of the white potato should be avoided. Research conducted at Cornell University in 1987 indicates that the skin of white potatoes contains toxic substances known as glycoalkaloids. Although the average person may be immune to these substances, they can adversely affect sensitive individuals to an alarming degree. In addition, Dr. Childers also concludes that the skins of white potatoes contain the highest amount of toxins. (Because yams or sweet potatoes are considered to be part of the morning glory family of plants and are not nightshades, they, as well as their skins, are permitted, as long as they are baked, boiled, or steamed and not fried.)

This is one area that conflicts with Cayce, for he highly recommended eating the skins of potatoes, but not the pulp, for the general public. We must remember, however, that we are dealing with psoriasis. Something that may have no affect on the average person can have a most serious effect in the psoriatic, thus the reason for my suggesting that my patients abstain from eating white potato skins as well as the pulp.

*Eggplant, peppers, and paprika.* These foods should not be consumed because of the highly toxic effect they have on the psoriatic. One of my patients, in particular, attributed the great improvement in his condition to the elimination of two favorite foods from his diet: eggplant and peppers. Hot, spicy foods, especially those made from nightshades, are to be totally avoided. (I am convinced that the high incidence of psoriasis in India is largely due to the country's hot, spicy diet.)

## Pizza—America's Favorite Food

It is well known that Americans love pizza. It has become more American than Mom's apple pie and is gaining in popularity all over the world. However, it is one of the worst food items the psoriatic can consume. Practically all of the ingredients that compose a pizza contribute to an over-acidic condition. For instance, the crust is usually made with white flour, tomato sauce (a nightshade) is spread on top of this, and the whole thing is covered by a thick layer of cheese. Peppers, also a nightshade, are a favorite pizza topping, as well as sausage, pepperoni, hot spices, and condiments. Put them all together and they are a nightmare for the psoriatic.

One patient related a story to me that is worth retelling. She was admitted into one of the major dermatological centers in New York City for a three-week stay in which PUVA therapy was her entire daily regimen. At the end of this period and at a cost of $20,000, she left the hospital with clear skin. It took exactly *one day* for the lesions to return in full bloom. As I notated her case history, I learned that diet, in general, was never a subject discussed at the center. In fact, she further related that if patients showed an interest in diet, their queries were simply made light of with the insinuation that diet is of no consequence. You can imagine my concern when she informed me that a party was held for all the psoriatics in her particular group at the end of her hospital stay. What kind of party? A pizza party, of all things!

Metaphorically speaking, if you eat pizza, you will soon resemble one. If I have not been convincing enough, I urge my readers to view the case of A.M., located in the photo section. As inconceivable as it may seem, her diet consisted of eating pizza, and practically no other foods every day. In her case, desperation forced her to seek alternative routes. Needless to say, I immediately eliminated pizza from her diet and placed her on the prescribed regimen. The dramatic result obtained speaks for itself.

In spite of what I have just stated regarding the consumption of pizza, I find no objection to my patients' eating an *occasional* slice of pizza, as long as it is prepared with natural, healthful foods such as whole-grain flours, fresh vegetables, chicken, turkey, low-fat/low-salt white cheeses, mild spices, and olive oil rather than the traditional types of ingredients such as white flour, tomato sauce, sausages, salami, peppers, pepperoni, whole-milk cheeses, anchovies, and hot spices.

## Salad Dressings and Olive Oil

Since fresh, green, leafy vegetable salads are an important part of the diet, the types of dressings to use are a major concern to most of my patients. More than any other type, I recommend fresh lemon juice or pure olive oil or a combination of the two. Peanut, canola, coconut, sunflower, sesame, soy or safflower oils, in sparing amounts, may be used as an alternative to olive oil. Plain low-fat yogurt or cottage cheese, cholesterol-free light mayonnaise, or commercial dressings that are 100 percent natural and free of additives and preservatives may also be used. *Avoid* all dressings containing wine or grain vinegar, tomatoes or other nightshades, and hot spices and seasonings. Take the time to read labels carefully. Apple cider vinegar may be added in small amounts provided that there is no adverse reaction.

Garnishes may include finely chopped hard-boiled egg yolks, feta cheese, tofu, chopped parsley and other fresh herbs, and mild spices and seasonings.

Olive oil carries more benefits than any other oil on the market. Recent studies classify olive oil as a monounsaturated fatty acid that reduces levels of artery-clogging cholesterol in the blood. Heart attacks are relatively rare in the Mediterranean countries such as Greece and Italy, because, according to Dr. Scott Grundy of the University of Texas Health Science Center in Dallas, olive oil is consumed in large quantities in both countries. Olive oil, in its natural state, is one of the most powerful, beneficial antioxidants known to man. If it is subjected to intense heat in cooking, however, it changes to what is called a *free radical,* which is very destructive to body cells. Use olive oil in its natural state as often as possible.

## Shellfish

My research suggests that all psoriatic and eczematous patients should completely avoid shellfish (lobster, shrimp, clams, oysters, crabs, scallops, snails, mussels, and so forth) and sauces made with shellfish. In addition, it should be noted that squid (calamari), even though it does not have a shell, is also classified as a shellfish. Although squid is low in fat, it contains the highest cholesterol-to-calorie ratio.

In my opinion, it is quite significant to note that shellfish contains high quantities of *purine bodies.* The end-product of the metabolism of purine compounds is uric acid. Elevated levels of uric acid are generally associated with gout. It has been noted that in some cases of psoriasis, secondary gout may be precipitated when the uric acid in the blood is elevated (hyperuricemia). Therefore it is not unreasonable to suspect the purine bodies contained in shellfish of being the culprit in triggering an allergiclike reaction in psoriasis and/or eczema patients.

## A Case in Point

I relate a story of one of my patients that borders on being a classic account as to whether shellfish plays a major role in controlling psoriasis in some people.

Mrs. E.G. had one of the most severe cases of psoriasis I have ever encountered. This woman had experienced virtually every known form of therapy over a twenty-five-year period. What little improvement took place was always short-lived.

After the usual indoctrination, Mrs. E.G. embarked on the regimen, and although it was painstakingly tedious to follow, it was not too long before she felt the beneficial effects of the new approach. I made it quite clear that it might take a year or more of constant adherence to the regimen. She agreed to stick with it. Improvement was slow but steady. She felt generally better, the scaling lessened, and the success of her efforts was clearly visible to her and her fellow employees.

As is often the case, she had to experiment for herself. She had to be convinced that diet played such an important role. She called to inform me of how great she was doing until "I had a few crabs, Dr. Pagano, and the next day, my back just broke out so badly that I couldn't believe it. Now I am convinced I can't break the diet." I asked her what she meant by a "few" crabs. She answered, "Well, maybe eight or ten at one sitting." Eight or ten, I advised her, are not just a few. Probably, if she had eaten one or two crabs, her body could have handled it, but eight or ten caused an allergic reaction that blossomed into a violent attack. This, I told her, was good, because she now knew that her system could not tolerate shellfish, at least not in the amount that she had eaten.

One of my cases, however, that of young B.M., indicates that with some people, even a small amount of shellfish is enough to cause a reaction. After this young woman had been completely clear of guttate psoriasis for two months, she ate one and one-half crabs. Her mother related that within three hours, lesions began to appear on her face, knees, and elbows. She immediately went on the Apple Diet and had an enema. The psoriasis began to clear overnight. A week before school started, her skin broke out again. Saffron tea fumes on her face and castor oil packs over her abdomen, along with Epsom salts baths, quickly brought the problem under control. It has now been several years since she responded so favorably and has remained clear ever since.

As in the previous case of E.G., B.M. no longer has to prove to herself that diet plays such an important role in controlling psoriasis. Both women know that they have only themselves to blame if their problem returns.

## Fish, Fowl, and Lamb

Fish, fowl (poultry), and lamb are the more readily digestible forms of animal protein and should, therefore, constitute part of the 20 percent of acid formers that the body needs daily.

### Fish

Fish is highly recommended because it is a major source of vitamins, minerals, and proteins. It is easily digestible and contains omega-3 fatty acids, which prevent cholesterol and other blood fats from building up on the walls of the arteries. These highly desirable fish oils are best obtained by eating fish rather than depending on supplements. The best seafood sources of omega-3 are fresh or canned salmon, sardines, and solid white albacore. Practically all species of fish are beneficial, especially the white-fleshed, cold-saltwater varieties. Some fish, however, do have a higher fat content, such as mackerel, bluefish, herring, and salmon; the darker and oilier the fish, the better. I advise my patients to consume such species as often as possible, in that they are known to be high in omega-3 fatty acids, which are now known to help heal the intestinal walls.

Fish may be broiled, grilled, baked, poached, or steamed—but not fried. A four- to six-ounce portion should be served at least four times a week. According to the American Medical Association, one fish meal a week can reduce the risk of sudden cardiac death by half. Fresh fish is always preferred; frozen fish, however, is acceptable. Always purchase "wild" varieties whenever possible, especially with regard to canned fish.

*Recommended:* Albacore (solid white), bass, bluefish, codfish, flounder, fluke, grouper, haddock, halibut, mackerel, mahimahi, perch, red snapper, salmon (wild is preferred over farm raised), sardines (fresh is preferred), scrod, sole, sturgeon, swordfish, trout, tuna, tilefish, and whitefish. (Sushi, made with brown rice and with fish taken from clean water, and sashimi may be eaten.)

*Not recommended*: Anchovies; pickled or creamed herring; lox; shellfish (clams, crabs, lobster, mussels, oysters, scallops, shrimp, squid, and so forth); sauces made from shellfish; coated fish (breaded or battered); fried or blackened (Cajun-style) fish; fish seasoned with hot spices or paprika or cooked with any other nightshades; any salted, dried, smoked, or pickled fish.

## Fowl (Poultry)

It goes without saying that fowl (poultry) in general is a primary source of protein throughout the world. Chicken breast, for example, according to the August 2005 Tufts University newsletter has a lot going for it as a source of animal protein: "Boneless, skinless chicken breasts offer great convenience and a good way to get protein (half your daily value in a three-ounce serving) without a lot of fat (three grams total, including just one gram of saturated fat) or calories (140, only 18 percent of them from fat). Broil, bake or grill—don't fry—to keep chicken a smart choice."

My suggestion to patients who consume chicken or other species of fowl is to choose certified organic, free-range, whenever possible, when purchasing poultry of any kind. Wild game is also more desirable than the commercial brands, to avoid antibiotics, hormones, and other possible harmful additives that are introduced into their food supply.

*Recommended*: Chicken, turkey, Cornish hens, and other types of nonfatty wild fowl (such as pheasant, guinea hens, and quail) are also recommended. Poultry may be prepared by any low-fat cooking method, such as broiling, steaming, poaching, baking, roasting, grilling, and boiling; it should not be fried. Any form of poultry may be cooked with the skin left on; however, the skin should always be removed before eating. According to Margaret Hoke, a supervisory nutritionist at the U.S. Department of Agriculture's Human Nutrition Information Service, there is no indication that fat migrates from the skin to the meat during the cooking process. Skinless white meat is preferred; the dark meat may be eaten on occasion. No more than a four- to six-ounce portion per serving, approximately twice a week, is suggested.

*Not recommended:* Poultry skin; dark meat (in cases of gout); fried or smoked poultry; any poultry that has not been thoroughly cooked; poultry that is battered, breaded, or heavily floured; deep-fried poultry; poultry that is highly seasoned or served with cream sauces, gravies, or hot spices; poultry garnished or cooked with paprika, tomatoes, peppers, white potatoes, or eggplant (in other words, nightshades).

## Lamb

Relatively speaking, lamb is perhaps the least popular of the red meats that are consumed in the United States. Lamb is the meat of young sheep less than a year old. Among the many nutrients attributed to lamb, zinc is one of the most valuable because zinc has a direct beneficial effect on the immune system. Since we are primarily concerned with enhancing the immune system, the opposite of what immuno-suppressive drugs do, lamb, if so desired, can play an important role in supplying the vital mineral zinc in the diet.

*Recommended:* The only red meat I suggest my patients consume is lamb, which is relatively easy to digest and is a high source of protein. No more than a four- to six-ounce serving, once or twice a week, is suggested. Lamb may be cooked by broiling, roasting, or grilling, but again, not fried, and should be served well done. All visible fat should be removed prior to cooking and before eating.

*Not recommended:* Any other red meat (beef, pork, veal, and all processed meats such as sausage, frankfurters, salami, ham, bologna, pastrami, corned beef, kielbasa, knockwurst, and so forth); visceral meats (heart, brains, kidneys, liver, sweetbreads); combining large portions of starches (bread, peas, corn, rice, winter squash, and so forth) with lamb.

Even though pork and pork products are not permitted, an *occasional* slice of very crisp bacon is allowed if a patient so desires.

## Dairy Products

Dairy products are generally permitted, provided that they are either nonfat or low-fat and low in sodium. Some of my patients, particularly those prone to arthritis, especially psoriatic arthritis, often experience adverse reactions when consuming any type of dairy product. Symptoms such as constipation, diarrhea, joint pains, stiffness, swelling of the hands, ankles, or feet, and indigestion indicate intolerance to this type of food. Should one or more of these reactions occur, refrain from consuming dairy products altogether. Alternate sources of calcium are foods such as tofu, dried figs, raisins, dates, celery, lettuce, turnip greens, kale, sesame seeds, and canned salmon and sardines, eaten with the bones.

I have often observed that a patient may either develop or already have intolerance to dairy foods at one point in time but, mysteriously, may not demonstrate any symptoms at another time. Therefore, the best route to take is to follow the dictates of one's own body. To reiterate, should a reaction occur, I suggest that one completely stop consuming any dairy product; if no reaction occurs, dairy products may be included in the daily diet in limited quantities and as long as they are low in fat and salt content.

*Recommended:* Milk (skim, 1%, low-fat, or nonfat; buttermilk; powdered milk; goat's milk, especially for those suffering from eczema; soy or almond milk [nondairy]), butter (sweet or unsalted; almond or sesame butter [nondairy]), cheese (low-fat, low-sodium, white cheese only), cottage cheese and cream cheese (plain, low-fat, low-sodium), sour cream and yogurt (plain, nonfat, or low-fat).

*Not recommended:* Any type of whole-milk dairy product; dairy products high in fat, sugar, or salt content; artificial dairy products; light, heavy, or whipped cream; ice cream and ice milk; orange and artificially colored cheese; salted, processed, or imitation butter; margarine made with hydrogenated oils; dairy products sweetened with cane sugars, artificial syrups, or chocolate flavorings; puddings and custards made with whole milk; dairy products (milk, cheese, or yogurt) combined with citrus fruits or their juices or stewed or dried fruit; consuming any dairy product that produces an allergic reaction.

## Grains

The advice I give my patients regarding grains is simple: Avoid white bread and all other products made with white flour. Whole-grain products are permitted but should not be overdone, since they are all acid formers, with the exception of millet and spelt, which are very close to being alkaline.

Some psoriatic patients suffer from a condition known as *celiac disease,* a gastrointestinal malfunction, without knowing it. It is an allergy toward gluten products. If this is the case, the patient is to avoid wheat, oats, rye, and barley products. If an improvement is seen within ten days, it is a positive sign that the patient is gluten intolerant. Further tests would then be warranted.

Whole grains, therefore, should be part of the 20 percent ratio of foods permitted in the daily diet. The bran (coverings) and the germ (seed) of the grain contain the vitamins, minerals, and protein. Whole grains act as a good eliminant due to their high fiber content.

Examples of permitted grains are oats, barley, millet, buckwheat, rye, groats (kasha), bran, wheat (whole, crushed, cracked, bulgur, wheat germ), corn and cornmeal, rice (brown and wild), and whole seeds (pumpkin, sesame, sunflower, flaxseed). (For best nutritional value, seeds should be soaked in water for twenty-four hours before eating. Seeds should be avoided altogether if a patient has diverticulosis.)

Products made from whole grains include breads, cereals (hot or cold), muffins, crackers, pretzels, pancakes and waffles, cookies, cakes, pie crusts, pasta, rice, and even pizza. Avoid bagels; they cause constipation.

*Recommended:* Breads and muffins made of whole grains including oats, bran, whole and cracked wheat, rye, pumpernickel, oat bran, and so forth. These products are best when toasted and, if desired, *lightly* spread with olive oil, unsalted (sweet) butter, low-fat margarine (made from cold-pressed oils), low-fat cream cheese, and/or a little honey or natural fruit preserves.

Cereal grains (high-fiber/whole-grain) such as bran, whole wheat (cracked, crushed), millet, oat bran, oats (rolled, cracked, and steel-cut), bulgur wheat, and so forth are acceptable.

You may also have hot or cold cereals such as Cream of Wheat, shredded wheat, puffed wheat, Ralston 100% Wheat Hot Cereal, Maltex, Wheatena, Nutri-Grain, seven-grain cereal, Uncle Sam Cereal, Total, and oatmeal. (Hot cereals should not be overcooked, as this will destroy the vitamin and mineral content.) Alkaline cereals are amaranth, millet, and quinoa.

*Additives may include:* Skim or low-fat milk, wheat germ, cinnamon, slivered or chopped almonds, a little honey, pure maple syrup or molasses (both sparingly). Also, any fruit (other than raw apples, bananas, melon, citrus, dried or stewed fruit) may be added, but in limited amounts. Strawberries are not permitted in cases of psoriatic arthritis.

Perhaps the most important basic rules to remember are: Do not combine citrus fruits or citrus juices with whole grains at the same meal, and avoid any whole-grain product if it creates an allergic reaction.

## Pasta

Pasta is a favorite food in many countries. There is no reason why the psoriatic cannot enjoy pasta dishes, provided the pasta is whole grain or vegetable in its makeup (not white-flour pasta).

*Recommended:* Jerusalem artichoke (sunchoke), carrot, spinach, corn, soy, egg, mung bean, whole wheat, and buckwheat noodles. Cellophane rice noodles are a good substitute for regular white-flour spaghetti, macaroni, and noodles. Newer products such as saffron noodles and parsley/garlic pasta are constantly finding their way onto the shelves of supermarkets as well as specialty gourmet food shops.

These pastas may be prepared with mild herbs and spices; fresh, steamed, or cooked vegetables (pasta primavera); pesto sauce (basil, garlic, olive oil, almonds, or pine nuts); or an olive oil–garlic sauce. A good low-carb pasta is Dreamfield's.

*Always avoid:* Sauces made from tomatoes, butter, cream, shellfish, clam sauce (white or red), and hot spices.

## Rice

Rice is a world staple. It is found throughout all corners of the earth. Its value in sustaining the human race, particularly in the Far East, is without equal.

There really is only one thing to remember about rice in cases of psoriasis, and that is to avoid eating white rice. Instead of white, polished rice, I advise my patients to consume only brown or wild rice. It must be remembered that rice, being a grain, is acid forming, so, once again, enjoy it, but not to excess. It may be eaten boiled or steamed but not fried.

*Recommended:* Whole-grain rice cakes make a good snack. Varieties include rye, sesame, buckwheat, and multigrain. Again, white rice cakes are to be avoided.

Toppings on rice cakes could include: honey (1 teaspoon); natural fruit jams, jellies, and preserves (1 teaspoon); low-fat white cheese (1 slice), low-fat ricotta or cottage cheese (1 teaspoon); white-meat turkey or chicken (1 slice), plain low-fat yogurt, or any noncitrus fruit.

My patients often ask about crackers, pretzels, and popcorn. I suggest unsalted matzos, Ry-Krisp, low-fat/unsalted saltines, unsalted wheat and oat bran crackers, unsalted whole-grain pretzels, and unsalted, unbuttered air-popped popcorn.

In general, therefore, the basic thing to remember about grains is to enjoy them in moderation. Choose only the whole-grain products, avoid the white-flour products, and do not mix cereals and citrus products at the same meal. If one abides by these simple rules, grains will not be a problem. In fact, they will add to the enjoyment and nutritional value of the daily diet.

## Sweets

It is of the utmost importance that psoriatic, psoriatic arthritic, and eczema sufferers eliminate most fats, white-flour products, and sugary sweets (sugary cereals, frostings, candy, regular or diet soda, and so forth) from their diet. There are, however, natural and nutritious substitutes that will satisfy the body's craving for sweets.

*For the sweet tooth:* Fresh fruit or fruit salads; dried, unsulphured tropical fruits; stewed or cooked fruits (figs, prunes, apricots, apples, and so forth); homemade applesauce or 100 percent natural store-bought applesauce; baked apple sweetened with honey, maple syrup, or a sprinkling of brown sugar and cinnamon; fruit juices (grape, pear, apricot, and papaya); Knox unflavored gelatin combined with diced fruit, water, and fruit juice; plain, organic, low-fat yogurt; low-fat frozen yogurt; fresh fruit sorbets; 100 percent natural frozen fruit bars; all-natural whole-grain cookies.

Honey, one of nature's most perfect foods, as well as pure maple syrup and molasses, is permitted, if consumed in small amounts. These sweeteners serve as an excellent topping for breads, muffins, and cereals.

Contrary to popular belief, carob is *not* a good substitute for chocolate. According to the Center for Science in the Public Interest, carob is saturated with fat and may be even more conducive to heart disease than beef fat.

Since sweets are generally acid formers, they should be selected carefully. The *natural* sweets derived mainly from fresh or dried fruits can supply the sugars necessary to form the alcohol needed for proper digestion and assimilation.

If, for any reason, these suggestions do not fulfill your craving for sweets, you may occasionally indulge in a *small* portion of a favorite dessert.

## Artificial Sweeteners

For several years, specific artificial sweeteners such as saccharin have been brought under the scrutiny of the FDA as possible cancer producers. The November 1985 edition of the *Journal of the American Medical Association* presented findings regarding this subject matter. The article clearly vindicated saccharin as a cancer producer and stated that the evidence does not support a link to cancer in humans. The report by the American Medical Association's Council on Scientific Matters further declared, "Available evidence indicates that . . . saccharin is not associated with an increased risk of bladder cancer." It further stated that "the AMA is not implying that it condones the use of saccharin." It did, however, support the sweetener's availability as a food additive.

In July 1985 the AMA concluded that the normal use of another artificial sweetener, aspartame, sold on the market as NutraSweet, was not associated with serious health problems. Reports have been filtering down, however, on the adverse effects that NutraSweet has had on some individuals, in the form of headaches, dizziness, and seizures, especially in teenagers. Only time and further research will settle this issue. In general, therefore, I do permit my patients to use artificial sweeteners, but only in minimal amounts. I always remind them that the ultimate effect artificial products have on the human body is still a controversial subject. Natural sweeteners, however, are now readily available to the consumer. The most popular are Splenda, stevia, fructose, and xylitol, a natural, low-glycemic sugar substitute. More on this subject is found in my cookbook, *Dr. John's Healing Psoriasis Cookbook . . . Plus!* available at www.psoriasis-healing.com.

# Beverages

Liquid intake, especially pure water, should be of primary interest to the psoriatic. The bathing of the cells, the flushing of the kidneys, the movements throughout the small and large intestines, and the chemical processes of the body are, to a great extent, if not completely, dependent on a healthy, fluid environment. It goes without saying that the type of liquid intake chosen should be relatively free of toxins, pollutants, destructive artificial additives, preservatives, colorings, or any other potentially harmful product. The optimum is to select those liquids that are cleansing and healthful and that enhance, rather than hinder, these vital body processes.

## Water

During the preliminary consultation with many of my new psoriasis patients, I am often amazed to find that they rarely, if ever, drink pure water daily. In fact, it is unusual to meet anyone who drinks more than one or two glasses a day. Most people feel that their daily water intake is adequately supplied through the foods they eat or by other liquids such as diet soda, alcohol, beer, coffee, or tea. Obviously, there are many individuals, without chronic skin conditions, whose bodies can apparently handle such an accumulation of toxins. In cases of psoriasis or eczema, however, such a violation can only aggravate an already overpolluted system.

I am not one to harp on rules, but if ever there was a rule that I insist be followed, especially for a psoriatic, it is this one: drink six to eight 8-ounce glasses of pure water a day, in addition to all other beverages consumed. As a matter of fact, I have found that patients suffering from psoriasis respond more readily when they make water their *only* drink (except for the teas), especially in the first few months of the regimen.

Water is not only convenient, inexpensive, and calorie-free, but it can also effectively curb your appetite. Whenever you are hungry, or before a meal, I suggest you drink a glass of water. Because water is tasteless, it can also help curb the desire for sweets and other beverages.

As an alternative to plain water, you may add the juice of four or five fresh lemons or limes to a gallon of spring, filtered, or bottled water. The water should then be refrigerated and consumed whenever desired. This will help the body processes in cleansing, lubrication, and alkalinity. (Refer to "The Importance of Water" in chapter 5.)

## Fruit and Vegetable Juices

Unsweetened fruit juices and vegetable juices are to be consumed as often as possible. If a rash occurs or the skin becomes sensitive due to drinking too much orange or grapefruit juice, drink less or eliminate it. All juices should be either freshly made or, if store-bought, purchased in a glass container or waxed carton. Avoid all canned juices.

A few drops to a quarter cup of lemon or lime juice should be added to a six- to eight-ounce glass of orange juice or grapefruit juice. Pure grape juice and other nutritious juices such as pineapple, pear, papaya, mango, and apricot are also recommended. Combinations of these juices are also suggested.

Vegetable juices as well as fruit juices are best freshly made in a home juicer. There is one major restriction regarding vegetable juices: avoid tomato juice and all juices that contain tomato. Occasionally adding a packet of Knox unflavored gelatin to a glass of fruit or vegetable juice will help to ensure maximum nutritional absorption.

Always keep in mind that consuming too much of any one food item, even if it is on the permitted list, can produce toxicity in the body. For instance, consuming too many carrots or drinking too much carrot juice can produce hypercarotenemia, bringing about pseudojaundice. An overabundance of fruit can raise the triglyceride level of the blood, which can cause a skin reaction. In other words, avoid extremes.

## Coffee

The debate over the effects coffee has on the human organism has been going on for more than fifty years. In 1986, scientific data was released to the public that indicated that people who consumed more than three cups of coffee per day were at risk of impairing their calcium absorption as well as developing heart disease. According to a study by the Johns Hopkins Medical School in Baltimore, anyone who drinks five or more cups of coffee a day has more than twice the risk of having heart problems than someone who drinks no coffee at all. This survey was conducted on one thousand men over a twenty-five-year period.

In October 1990, however, new findings published in the *New England Journal of Medicine* completely refuted the previous findings, revealing that a study of more than forty-five thousand men found no evidence that coffee boosts the risk of heart disease or stroke.

What is one to do? Follow the experts, and you find yourself in a state of confusion. Do whatever you please, and you may jeopardize your health. Consequently, I feel that using common sense is the answer. I suggest that those of my patients who feel a need to drink coffee consume no more than three cups of black decaffeinated coffee per day, in other words, without milk, cream, or sugar. Those who have little desire for coffee should eliminate it altogether. It seems to me that the question here is not whether coffee in itself is harmful, but rather how much is consumed. An unreasonable amount can lead not only to physical reactions but to mental reactions as well.

### A Case in Point

Mr. A.G. came into my office suffering from a rather severe degree of psoriasis, which he had had for twenty years. The primary areas involved were across his upper back, his shoulders, and down each arm. What disturbed him most, however, was the severity of the disease throughout his hands. His profession involved being in close contact with the public. Because of his embarrassment, he would take whatever measures were necessary to avoid exposing his hands.

Rarely have I had such a cooperative patient. Without question or complaint, A.G. did everything that was required. Although the progress was slow, it was steady. In a few months, his back, his shoulders, and most of his upper arms cleared up nicely—however, the tops of his hands showed no change. He noticed that during the week, the lesions of his hands would not be so inflamed; yet on weekends, they would flare up to an intolerable degree. This pattern repeated itself every week.

We sat down and tried to figure out the reason for this recurrence. Was there something that A.G. was doing, or perhaps not doing, that caused this adverse reaction to occur only on weekends? There was: he drank too much coffee. During the week when he was busy working as a traveling salesman, he would drink seven to ten cups of coffee a day.

On weekends, when he was an auctioneer, which placed him under a great deal of stress, he would drink as many as sixteen or seventeen cups a day. There was no need to look any further. I reminded A.G. that although black coffee was permitted on the diet, drinking sixteen cups a day was utterly ridiculous. The maximum that I allowed was three cups per day. A.G. decided not only to cut down on his coffee intake on weekends but to refrain from drinking it altogether. He proved to me that when he made up his mind to do something, he did it.

Results were not immediate. Three weeks passed without any apparent change in his condition. I was ready to give up the idea that coffee was the culprit, when a change began to take place. The remaining lesions on his lower arms began to dry up. He began to feel better in general, with his energy level greatly improving. Most important of all were the changes that occurred in his hands. The irritation on the tops of his hands was hardly visible. He and I were now convinced that the excessive amount of coffee that he had been drinking on weekends was the primary reason for the flare-ups.

Although three cups of coffee per day are allowed on the diet, after eliminating coffee altogether, several of my patients reported a marked improvement in the condition of their skin. As a substitute for coffee, some patients drink a cup of hot water with the juice of a lemon or lime, which seems to satisfy them.

## Herbal Teas

The teas involved in helping to heal psoriasis and eczema are natural herbal teas that affect the internal cleansing process and aid in the restoration of the intestinal walls. Most herbal teas do not contain caffeine, theobromide, or tannin, which are potentially harmful ingredients that can lead to nervousness, insomnia, rapid heartbeat, and disruption of blood-sugar levels. Popular commercial teas, however, do contain these unhealthy elements and should, therefore, be avoided by the psoriatic.

The most beneficial herbal teas are American yellow (not Spanish) saffron tea and slippery elm bark powder tea. Discussion of these teas and their preparation appears in chapter 7.

## Supplemental Herbal Teas

Other herbal teas may include watermelon seed tea, chamomile, mullein, and decaffeinated green or black tea. Oolong tea has been cited as being very helpful in cases of eczema.

## Milk

Generally, milk is hard to digest and can be constipating. It produces a great deal of mucus. Because of this, athletes training in sports where good respiration is essential may benefit by eliminating whole milk from their diet. Milk is not considered to be an acid former; therefore it is included in the diet, but only in the form of skim or low-fat milk and milk in its predigested form, such as low-fat buttermilk and low-fat yogurt. Soy and goat's milk have been found to be more easily tolerated by patients with eczema.

## Carbonated Drinks

Carbonated soft drinks are saturated with sugars, preservatives, artificial flavorings, and colorings. In spite of the fact that regular and diet sodas contain these known detrimental ingredients, they are the most popular beverages consumed by the public. Since purification of the blood is the keynote in the healing of psoriasis, these drinks should be viewed as poison to all psoriatics. As discussed in an earlier chapter, the liver is perhaps the most active filtering gland of the body. It must be in peak condition, without blockages or hindrances of any kind to function properly. The excessive consumption of soda has such a destructive effect on the liver that some authorities feel that even one glass a day is too much.

Dr. S. H. Hutner, speaking at the University of Massachusetts, stated that "cirrhosis (disease) of the liver may as often affect soft-drink addicts as alcoholics." He theorizes that the "empty calories" in sugary sodas make people cut down on their consumption of wholesome foods, which produces a protein deficiency resulting in cirrhosis of the liver. The standard treatment for this condition is to place the patient on a high-protein, low-carbohydrate diet with vitamin supplements and to eliminate all soft drinks.

As a substitute for soft drinks, I recommend drinking an occasional glass of cold naturally carbonated water, such as Perrier, San Pellegrino,

Saratoga water, or plain seltzer water (not club soda). These can be served over ice with fresh lemon or lime juice added. Not only is this cleansing to the system, but it is also thirst quenching, delicious, and satisfying. Many of my patients have even found this to be the solution to social drinking.

## Alcoholic Beverages

Of the sacrifices that a psoriatic must make, for some the elimination of alcohol is the most difficult, especially if the patient is a "drinker." If I find early on in my course of treatment that a patient is unwilling to accept the fact that he or she must avoid hard liquor in any form, I have no qualms in advising against further treatment.

Some years ago, a physician referred a psoriatic patient to me. She was most receptive to my suggestions and apparently followed through on all that was required of her. After only a few weeks, her psoriasis cleared up considerably; however, I never saw her again. Months went by before I met with the doctor who originally referred her to me. I informed him of this patient's negligence in continuing her treatments. He nodded his head in an understanding manner and said, "John, you didn't fail, she was responding beautifully—but she simply could not give up her dry martinis. She was just too embarrassed to tell you."

In cases of psoriasis and eczema, it is extremely important that alcohol, in all its forms, including beer, be totally eliminated. The only leeway that I allow my patients regarding alcohol is drinking an occasional glass of dry red or white wine. No more than two to four ounces is permitted with dinner or with a slice of dark bread late in the afternoon. The combination of wine, especially red wine, and brown bread is a powerful blood builder, according to the Cayce works. Taken in this manner, they are considered a "food." Wine, in itself, contains iron and plasm, which can benefit the system. For those who prefer white wine, I suggest a spritzer (half white wine and half seltzer with a slice of lemon over ice). Again, this is permitted only on occasion and should not become too much of a habit. A word of caution: If a patient is on any kind of medication or suffers from gout, wine is not permitted under any circumstances.

## "Doctor, Can I Cheat?"

A question that often arises is whether you can cheat on the diet. The answer is that some can get away with it, whereas others cannot. For most, it is unwise to break the diet during the first few months of the prescribed regimen. I encourage people to remain on the diet until they are clear of all lesions. After this has been accomplished, you can slowly add to the diet certain types of foods that were once enjoyed. If an unfavorable reaction begins to occur, that is, a recurrence of skin eruptions, you should immediately revert back to the recommended diet for a longer period of time. The deciding factor is whether the body is now capable of filtering out and removing toxins formed by acid-producing foods.

## Expect Weight Loss

The dietary suggestions contained herein offer an added benefit that is generally welcomed by most patients: a *healthy* weight loss. Many psoriatics carry ten or more pounds of excess baggage in the form of accumulated fat. When they hear that they can and will lose weight on this diet, they are encouraged by knowing that they have an excellent opportunity to rid themselves not only of psoriasis, but also of their unwanted pounds. Loss of excess weight has become such a consistent finding that when no weight loss is evident, it is a strong indication to me that the patient is not adequately adhering to the diet, even though he or she may try to deny it.

Some people become alarmed when friends or relatives become overly concerned about their obvious weight loss. Usually, these well-meaning friends are simply unaccustomed to seeing a svelte figure appear before them. More often than not, a person on this diet feels better than ever, has an abundance of vitality, and is able to fit into stylish clothes, which, in itself, enhances his or her self-esteem.

I advise those who feel there is too much of a weight loss simply to eat more of the permitted foods listed in the "80 percent" category—that is, fruits, vegetables, and their juices—without overindulging themselves. It should be noted that even though it is important to be conscious of the types of foods consumed, equal emphasis should be placed on the quantity and the size of the portions eaten, as well as the proper combination of foods. All of these factors determine the effect that foods have on the system. Those following the diet should never feel hungry. If they do, it is simply because they are not consuming enough of the body-building foods.

## Being Flexible

As important as it is to adhere to the diet as closely as possible, it should be maintained with a certain amount of flexibility. The entire dietary concept should not become an irritating, restrictive chore because of an attempt to be overly precise regarding every food item listed. Allowing for an expected number of failures, adherence to the basic dietary suggestions for a long enough period usually brings about satisfactory results.

Although there are certain restrictions, such as fatty foods and the nightshades, most of the diet can be followed and adhered to with a certain amount of leeway and flexibility without affecting the overall result. I see no harm in occasionally satisfying a desire for a specific food after being on the diet for a few weeks, as long as it is not over-done and there is no adverse reaction.

The feelings of restriction will be less intense and not as frustrating if one is determined to make the diet interesting, tasty, and as creative as possible. There are many nutritious-recipe cookbooks on the market today that contain helpful suggestions and recipes that utilize the allowed foods. Once you are familiar with these preparations, the entire procedure will become simpler, more appealing, and consequently, more enjoyable.

In 2000, I completed my cookbook, which contains over three hundred recipes and much additional health-related information designed for the psoriatic-eczematous patient. *Dr. John's Healing Psoriasis Cookbook . . . Plus!* now sells all over the world and makes living a healthy lifestyle much easier, more pleasant, and more effective not only for the patient but for the cook. The cookbook may be ordered online at my Web site, www.psoriasis-healing.com.

## Overeating

To obtain successful results with the regimen, it is important to consume only moderate-size portions of the foods permitted. There have been some cases where overindulging in these foods has proven to be the reason for a delayed beneficial reaction.

It is not uncommon to find that some people who fail to respond to the regimen do so because they consume *too much* of the foods recommended, especially where meats and sweets are concerned. Consequently, as mentioned previously, there should always be a conscious awareness of the quantity of food consumed. Simply because a food item is permitted does not grant a person license to overindulge.

I recall that one patient who had been advised to eat a *few* almonds a day proceeded to consume a *full pound* of nuts in one evening. His reasoning was that because almonds appeared on the recommended list of foods, the more he ate, the better! With still another patient who did not respond after maintaining the diet for several months, just cutting back on the *quantity* of allowed foods caused not only a desirable weight loss, but cleared up all of her psoriatic lesions at the same time. As the fat diminished, a sense of well-being took place, apparently because of the relief that losing the extra weight brought to her heart, lungs, liver, and skin. Therefore, when there is a choice of eating more or less, always eat less.

## Food Allergies

Even though specific foods appear in the diet, some may not always have an agreeable effect. With some individuals, there are permitted foods that may possibly cause an allergic reaction. The Apple Diet, if you remember from chapter 5, is one of the most effective ways to cleanse the body of internal toxins. The vast majority of my patients have had no difficulty maintaining this diet for three days. However, one of my patients advised me that eating any kind of apple could cause such a violent allergic reaction in the form of throat constriction that it might possibly endanger her life. Even having an apple touch her lips resulted in swelling so severe that she could barely open her mouth. Obviously, the Apple Diet was not for her. In another instance, a patient was able to eat all the carrots she wanted but could not touch them because her fingers would blister and break out in a rash. Similar reactions have been known to occur in some patients after consuming dairy products, citrus fruits and juices, and products made of wheat. Patients should avoid all foods that they know will have a detrimental effect on them, even though they are noted as permitted on the dietary list contained herein.

Food allergies are more common and far-reaching than formerly understood. Identifying personal food allergies does not fall within the scope of this book. As a point of reference, the following foods account for the majority of food allergies: milk, eggs, fish (bass, flounder, cod), crustacean shellfish (crab, lobster, shrimp), tree nuts (almonds, walnuts, pecans), peanuts, wheat, and soybeans.

For those interested, two allergy/sensitivity tests are available: (1) the cytotoxic test, capable of identifying up to 250 foods or additives, and (2) the leukocyte antigen sensitivity test (LAST), considered by many to be more thorough and accurate than the cytotoxic test. These tests should be performed only under qualified medical supervision.

## Vitamins and Minerals

The question of whether vitamin supplements are necessary in the management of psoriasis is often asked by patients and physicians alike. My research suggests that they play only a minor role, provided that a patient adheres to the dietary regimen. Necessary vitamins and minerals obtained from their natural state, that is, from foods such as fruits and vegetables and their juices, far surpasses those obtained from synthetic, manufactured sources. Nevertheless, there are instances when they may be of some value, if only from a psychological point of view.

The vitamins and minerals most frequently associated with psoriasis are vitamins A and D, as well as the B vitamins. According to Melvyn R. Werbach, MD, in his classic account *Nutritional Influences on Illness,* during a ten-year experimental psoriasis study, 118 out of 155 patients responded with purified granulated soya phosphatides. Crude lecithin, 3 to 6 grams daily, was also given, in addition to small amounts of vitamins A, D, $B_1$, $B_2$, $B_6$, and calcium pantothenate. When using vitamin $D_3$ with a control base, applied topically, five out of five patients showed "remarkable improvement." Other sources indicate that similar results have been obtained by using vitamin E topically. I found it particularly noteworthy that Dr. Werbach also cited in another experimental study that six out of six patients improved on *elimination diets.*

In short, vitamin supplements may prove beneficial in some cases and generally pose no threat to the patient. A person should, however, first consult with a licensed health practitioner before embarking on a therapeutic regimen of vitamins, whether they are administered systemically or topically.

## Dietary Supplements

The popularity of dietary supplements, especially natural ones, has recently grown to an all-time high. Throughout history across all major cultures and civilizations, natural herbs were once the only means of cure or relief for disease. Then came the pharmaceutical companies—need I say more? The rest is history—or current events!

It has been postulated that there is a natural herbal remedy for every disease known to man. The validity of that statement is not for me to say, but this subject is addressed in the next chapter.

Today, certain herbal remedies are associated with the healing of psoriasis. In 1999, *Reader's Digest* published an extensive book *The Healing Power of Vitamins, Minerals, and Herbs,* which included an impressive discourse on psoriasis as well as eczema. It contains perhaps the most concise, detailed list of supplements available to the psoriatic patient. Here, by permission, I reproduce the precise chart as it was published in 1999. It is the most noteworthy list (which includes dosages) that I have ever encountered:

## Supplement Recommendations

| | |
|---|---|
| **Essential fatty acids** | **Dosage:** 1,000 mg fish oil 3 times a day; 1 tbsp. (14 grams) flaxseed oil each morning. |
| | **Comments:** People with diabetes should take less than 2,000 mg of fish oils a day; higher doses can worsen blood sugar control. |
| **Grape seed extract** | **Dosage:** 100 mg twice a day. |
| | **Comments:** Standardized to contain 92%-95% proanthocyanidins. |
| **Alpha-lipoic acid** | **Dosage:** 150 mg each morning. |
| | **Comments:** Can be taken with or without food. |
| **Vitamin A** | **Dosage:** 25,000 IU a day for 1 month, then 10,000 IU daily. |
| | **Comments:** Women who are pregnant or considering pregnancy should not exceed 5,000 IU a day. |
| **Zinc/Copper** | **Dosage:** 30 mg zinc and 2 mg copper a day. |
| | **Comments:** Add copper only when using zinc longer than 1 month. |
| **Milk thistle** | **Dosage:** 150 mg twice a day. |
| | **Comments:** Standardized to contain at least 70% silymarin. |

**Some dosages may be supplied by supplements you are already taking.**

Reprinted with permission from *The Healing Power Of Vitamins, Minerals, And Herbs*, copyright © 1999 by The Reader's Digest Association, Inc., Pleasantville, New York, www.rd.com.

In cases of eczema, the chart indicates that most of the same measures are called for in cases of eczema (atopic dermatitis), except for the addition of a cream that contains chamomile or licorice (called glycyrrhetinic acid cream). These herbs reduce skin inflammation and can be surprisingly soothing when applied three or four times a day directly to the lesions.

## Out of Sight, Out of Mind

One of the most effective measures that one can take in making the diet easier to follow is simply to buy only those foods that are recommended and avoid purchasing those that are not. The refrigerator and kitchen cabinets should be well stocked with these foods at all times.

Obviously, if you live alone, this is easier to do, but families, spouses, and roommates who have followed this diet along with the patient have often commented to me that it was beneficial to them as well. They not only felt better generally and lost excess weight, but they were helping their friend or loved one at the same time by encouraging him or her to maintain the diet.

## When Dining Out

There are many people who, because of their profession, occupation, or lifestyle, eat many or most of their meals in restaurants. Even so, it is not impossible to have your food specially prepared when eating out. Currently, there are many restaurants that are conscious of individual preferences and will gladly accommodate their patrons by preparing foods according to the customer's wishes. I encourage people to take advantage of this and make their desires known.

I tell my patients to do the following when dining out:

- Select foods that are steamed, broiled, stir-fried, poached, baked, grilled, or cooked in their own juices.
- Order fish, nonfatty fowl, or lamb. Do not order beef, pork, veal, or shellfish.
- Avoid ordering fried, blackened, buttered, creamed, au gratin, or breaded foods and those with rich sauces.
- Ask the waiter how a dish is prepared.
- Request that the chef avoid buttering before broiling, that salad dressing be served on the side, and that low-fat cheese be substituted for high-fat.
- Trim off all visible fat on meats and poultry before eating. Remove the skin from poultry before eating (it may be cooked with the skin on).
- Select whole-grain breads and bread sticks, rather than high-fat croissants, corn bread, or biscuits.
- Order à la carte whenever possible so that you may be more selective.
- To satisfy a sweet tooth, order fresh fruit, low-fat frozen yogurt, naturally sweetened fruit ices, or any other type of low-fat dessert.

- When dining in Italian restaurants, order menu items described as *affogato* (steamed or poached).
- In Chinese restaurants, order steamed vegetable dishes, poached fish dishes, and steamed poultry dishes. Avoid eating beef, pork, or shellfish dishes, and foods prepared with MSG (monosodium glutamate).
- Avoid ordering hot, spicy dishes. Select the more lightly seasoned entrées.
- Always order a large green leafy salad, such as a garden salad, but avoid eating any nightshades. The preferred salad dressing is olive oil and lemon juice.

# A Mini Review

My experience with psoriasis leads me to the unquestionable conclusion that it is what you *avoid* putting into the body, combined with what you *flush out,* that helps the psoriatic patient the most. Remember, psoriasis is caused by a toxic buildup. Therefore, get rid of the accumulated toxins and don't put any more in.

These toxins come primarily from the food you eat. It may be good food and expensive food, but it is the *wrong* food.

## Food Items to Consume

It should come as a pleasant surprise that since the publication of the first printing of this book, in 1991, many nutritional facts have been established that reinforce the value of the dietary measures first described in my original text. For example:

- Green leafy vegetables, permitted fresh fruits, and fish (not shellfish) are the most valuable foods to consume. (Refer to appendix A for more details.)
- It is vital to consume plenty of water. Coffee, soft drinks, beer, and regular commercial tea are not good substitutes for pure water. To drink more water than air, drink through a straw, rather than from a glass or a bottle. (*Note:* Nutritionists now believe that cold water is more readily absorbed by the body than water at room temperature.)

- Never drink while you are eating. If you do, your body's signals for enzymes get confused. Enzymes break down food for proper absorption. If they are washed out, proper digestion is impaired. Water should be consumed a half hour before eating and a half hour after, not during the meal.

- If you have kidney disease or congestive heart disease or use a diuretic, consult with your medical doctor before increasing water intake.

- The benefits of eating more fruits and vegetables far outweigh any risks from exposure to pesticides, according to a panel sponsored by the Canadian National Consumer Institute (*The Record,* May 4, 1998). I advocate washing fresh vegetables and fruits thoroughly before eating, and I prefer them to be organically grown whenever possible.

- The most valuable green leafy vegetable for the psoriatic (or anybody) is romaine lettuce. According to the Cayce works, green leafy vegetables such as romaine lettuce are blood purifiers. Always wash lettuce and greens before eating.

- A delicious, nutritious vegetable-juice combination is to juice a bunch of carrots, one or two stalks of celery, and a small- to medium-size beet.

- A wonderful, popular cup of tea is a mixture of green tea, a teaspoon of honey, and a teaspoon of ginseng. Many people drink it in place of coffee in the morning.

- Sweet potatoes (a morning glory, not a nightshade) are considered to be one of the most beneficial of all tuber vegetables for anyone, especially in cases of psoriasis and eczema.

- I do not hesitate to state that the most important supplements for the psoriasis-eczema patient are omega-3 fish oils and flaxseed oil. Their value is found in their action on the intestinal wall mucosa (inner lining). As does slippery elm, they help repair the compromised intestinal wall, which is where we want to focus our attention. Other oils, such as cat's claw, evening primrose, and olive, possess the same attributes. Recently there have been reports from various sources regarding the beneficial effects of organic extra-virgin coconut oil (or at least natural coconut oil) used both internally and externally.

Obtaining omega-3 from eating fish itself is much preferred. The species that carry the greatest quantity of omega-3 are the more fatty, oily fish such as Atlantic salmon, mackerel, bluefish, tuna, fresh sardines, halibut, and herring. The 1998 NIH report on omega-3 lists fish, spinach, and squash as the best sources.

## The Deadly Seven

Most of us with any kind of ailment feel we must take something in order to get well. We have been raised that way. In many cases, of course, this is true, but does it ever occur to us that it is what we are *taking in* (ingesting) that is causing the problem? The antidote, of course, is to *stay away from such items.*

I call them the "Deadly Seven." They are seven things that over the years I have observed to be the culprits when dealing with psoriasis and eczema. Remember, it may very well be that your entire healing will depend on what you stay away from.

1. Saturated fats—such as red and processed meats
2. Nightshades—especially tomatoes, peppers, and hot spices
3. Too many sweets
4. Smoking
5. Alcohol
6. Junk food (for adults as well as children)
7. Fried foods

You would be surprised at how many people have reported to me that staying away from one or more of these items resulted in improvement within a matter of days. Study them, write them down, memorize them; then do yourself a favor and stay away from them!

## The Glorious Seven

Here are the winners, the food items that can spell success:

1. Fresh water, six 8-ounce glasses a day (you may add fresh lemon or lime juice).
2. Vegetables, green leafy in particular, as well as tubers. The ratio of these vegetables should be three that grow *above* the ground to one that grows *below.* Keep the acid-alkaline balance. Vegetables and fruit should be 80 percent of the daily diet.

3. Fresh fruit—they are the body cleansers. They are to be avoided, however, in cases of candida and yeast-fungi overgrowth.

4. Fish, fowl, and lamb, as animal protein. (Vegetarians should consider that brown rice and beans combine to make a complete protein.) These should constitute 20 percent of the daily diet.

5. Probiotics (yogurt, kefir) with active cultures.

6. Olive oil, garlic, and lemon juice, especially in cases of candida.

7. Whole-grain breads only—but not too much, as they are acid forming.

Remember to read labels and pick products with the lowest count of carbohydrates (which convert to sugar) and sugar content. This may seem hard for some people to do. It's a matter of where you place your priorities. Do you want to get well or not? The answer to that determines your future in matters of health.

## Final Comments

Common sense must be exercised when following any nutritional regimen. To reiterate, if a particular food does not agree with you, even if it appears on the permitted-food list, it is to be avoided. If feelings of weakness or hunger are present, simply eat more of the body-building foods, but never to the point of being gluttonous. In short, discipline should be maintained in the *quantity* as well as the *quality* (type) of food consumed.

It has become obvious by now that select foods play a most significant role in healing psoriasis. The scientific community must eventually acknowledge the role that nutrition plays in skin diseases. Additional nutritional advice I offer my patients can be found in appendix A, along with a seven-day sample menu and several recipes found in appendix B.

Psoriatics the world over should heed the wisdom of Hippocrates, the father of medicine: "Let your food be your medicine—let your medicine be your food."

# CHAPTER 7

# Herbal Teas

When I was a boy, I was fascinated by the adventures of Tarzan in the famous stories by Edgar Rice Burroughs. I was particularly in awe of Tarzan's ability to heal the injured and ill with herbal medicines. The fact that Tarzan was able to cure internal and external ailments by extracting juices from various herbs and applying them directly to a wound or administering them orally rang true for me, for reasons I could not explain.

The Tarzan stories are fiction, of course, but are the methods of this primitive jungle physician so far-fetched? When you stop to think about it, all we have in this plane of existence, from a physical point of view, is derived from the earth. Herbs and herbal teas have been used for healing since the dawn of human history, and most of our modern drugs are still derived from plants. Our medicines today typically come in capsule form, carefully measured and attractively packaged, but they still have their origins in nature.

Commercial teas often contain caffeine, theobromine, and tannin, all of which are potentially harmful to the body. Taken at high potencies or in large quantities, they can lead to nervousness, insomnia, rapid heartbeat, and disruption of blood-sugar levels. In contrast, most herbal teas do not contain these potentially harmful ingredients, and some of these teas are very helpful in clearing psoriasis. Five specific herbs are recommended for this purpose. These herbs are (1) American yellow saffron, (2) slippery elm (in the form of ground bark powder or as capsules or lozenges), (3) chamomile, (4) mullein, and (5) water-melon seed tea.

Oolong tea has been recommended by some dermatologists for relief in cases of eczema. A study of more than a hundred patients reported in the Archives of Dermatology (January 2001) showed that drinking a liter of oolong tea daily could markedly decrease inflammation and itching.

I advise my patients to persist in taking the herbal teas as directed, and to have confidence that by doing so, they will be taking a major step in the alleviation of psoriasis.

*Note:* The herbal teas mentioned in this chapter are available at most well-supplied health food stores, or they may be ordered through the product suppliers listed in appendix D.

## Saffron Tea

The saffron called for in cases of psoriasis is the American yellow saffron (*Carthamus tinctorius*), not the "true" or Spanish saffron (*Crocus sativus*), which is grown not only in Spain but also in western Asia, France, Austria, and Iran. Most people would probably be shocked at the cost of Spanish saffron, which sells for at least $25 an ounce. This is because it takes about seventy-five thousand flowers to make one pound. Its value was known even in the time of Solomon, three thousand years ago, when it was used as a dye, in scented salves, and as an aromatic placed in the Greek halls and courts and in the Roman baths. Today, because of its expense, it is seldom used except for certain medicinal purposes and (primarily) as a flavoring in certain dishes.

American yellow saffron, often substituted for the Spanish variety, is produced mostly in the United States, England, and the countries surrounding the Mediterranean Sea. For the psoriatic, it is better than the Spanish saffron and only one-tenth of the price.

Saffron tea is the kind most frequently prescribed for a variety of ailments, not just psoriasis. The major ailments for which saffron tea is considered beneficial include psoriasis, lacerations, eliminations, incoordination of assimilations and eliminations, toxemia, and ulcers. From this list we can safely assume that saffron acts on the stomach and intestines and helps alleviate skin ailments caused by a malfunction in the alimentary canal.

Note that slippery elm and American yellow saffron herbal teas are not recommended for women who are pregnant or who expect to become pregnant, as they have been implicated in causing miscarriage, but only in rare cases.

## Preparation of Saffron Tea

Place about a quarter teaspoon of saffron tea in a cup, then pour boiling water over it and stir. Cool, strain, and drink. This should be made fresh each time it is taken. Note that saffron tea is best taken at night, just before retiring. Some patients report that they enjoy having a few cups during the day as well. The most beneficial effects of the tea are that it flushes out the liver and kidneys, increases perspiration, and promotes healing of intestinal lesions. Saffron tea has also been called an intestinal antiseptic. It should be regarded as a valuable part of the therapeutic regimen. This tea is to be taken consistently until the skin is clear, or at least five days a week, and then periodically to keep the "passageways" cleansed for proper elimination.

Saffron water is a variant of saffron tea that can be helpful in severe cases of psoriasis. The idea is to have some saffron in all of the patient's drinking water. Although saffron water is not as concentrated as the tea, its cleansing effect is without equal.

To make saffron water, boil one gallon of pure water and add one teaspoon of American yellow saffron tea; allow the mixture to steep for twenty minutes. This will be just enough to give the water a yellowish tinge. When the water cools, strain it and pour it into a glass or porcelain container or the original gallon jug the water came in, and refrigerate. This is to be used as drinking water whenever desired. I recommend at least two to four glasses of saffron water a day. This may be considered part of the suggested daily intake of six to eight glasses of drinking water. In time, the cleansing effect of the saffron water will bring about beneficial results, provided all other rules of the regimen are followed.

In the event that swelling occurs in the ankles and lower legs, cut water consumption (including saffron water) in half, as this condition indicates water retention from consuming too much liquid. If this happens, consult a medical doctor about the use of a diuretic to relieve the swelling.

Occasionally, you may develop the sensation of needing to urinate even when the bladder has recently been emptied. This can be attributed to the cleansing effect of the saffron tea. After a period of time, in flushing out the kidneys, the tea causes a constant flow of urine into the bladder. The person begins urinating more often than he or she is used to, causing the inner lining of the bladder to wear down somewhat, especially in the area of the sphincter trigone at the bottom of the bladder. This, in turn, causes stimulation of the stretch fibers, giving the sensation that you have to urinate even when it is not necessary. If this occurs, stop drinking the tea until the sensation passes.

Saffron vapor can be useful in dealing with psoriasis on the face. Although the condition appears less frequently on the face and the hands, there are many cases in which psoriasis breaks out in these areas. This can cause considerable anxiety in the patient because these areas are highly visible. Exposure of the head and hands to the rays of the sun undoubtedly helps keep these areas relatively clear of the lesions, but when this is not enough, some of my patients have succeeded in clearing facial psoriasis by steeping some saffron or chamomile tea in a basin of hot water, then placing a towel over the head and leaning over the basin, allowing the steam to gently stimulate the skin. (The procedure is similar to using Vicks VapoSteam to break up a cold in the head.)

One patient in particular had excellent results when, after the steam, she rubbed castor oil into the lesions and left it on overnight. As early as the next morning, after washing her face with Cuticura soap, she saw a noticeable improvement. However, real clearing comes from the generalized internal cleansing of the body. This proved to be true in this case when the patient realized that the steam treatment was, at best, only temporary. She then drank a half gallon of saffron water over a period of a few hours. Urination was extremely frequent because of this measure, but within one day her face was practically 100 percent clear. She attributes this remarkable result to the large quantity of saffron water she consumed. A general flushing of the liver and the kidneys took place and helped drain the body of accumulated toxins. Today, this patient's face is always as clear as she wants it to be.

American yellow saffron tea is one of the most difficult teas to find, even in well-supplied health food stores. I advise my patients to contact Baar Products or the Heritage Store (see appendix D) and order it directly from them.

# Slippery Elm Bark Tea

The Chinese have long enjoyed the many benefits of slippery elm. They consider it one of nature's most excellent demulcents and nutritives and employ it for its ability to absorb foul gases in the body; for its gentle, soothing action in cases of enteritis (inflammation of the intestinal tract) and colitis (inflammation of the large bowel); and because its soothing, mucilaginous nature makes bowel evacuation easier and more effective.

From these accounts, as well as the Chinese influence, we can conclude that the slippery elm acts as a protective coating along the inner lining of the upper and lower intestinal tract. Not only can this prevent seepage of toxins, it also helps in healing the thin, porous intestinal walls and aids in evacuation.

## Preparation of Slippery Elm Bark Tea

Place about a quarter to one-half of a teaspoon of slippery elm bark powder in a cup of warm water. Stir and let stand about fifteen minutes before drinking. Do not let it stand beyond thirty minutes, as it may become rancid. This mixture is taken in the early morning, at least one-half hour before breakfast, if possible, for the first ten days of the regimen. It is then reduced to every other day, except in severe cases, until the skin condition clears. Most people have no problem swallowing the slippery elm drink, but if it is difficult to get down, adding ice to the mixture may help.

Slippery elm bark is also available and may be chewed. For some people this is no problem; most find it not only difficult to do, but unsightly as well. A more palatable and convenient alternative is to purchase Thayer's Slippery Elm Lozenges in a health food store or a well-supplied drugstore. Taking a few of these a day usually serves the same purpose.

The importance of taking saffron and slippery elm, especially in severe or stubborn cases of psoriasis, cannot be overemphasized. These herbal teas affect the gastric flow throughout the stomach and stimulate the walls of the intestinal tract to bring about healing of the distressed areas.

Remember, our approach to alleviating psoriasis is primarily based on diet, healing the intestinal walls, and ensuring adequate evacuation. Slippery elm bark powder, as a tea or a chewable lozenge, taken regularly, is a vital part of this healing process, and I consider it mandatory, with one important exception: as noted previously, women who are pregnant or who expect to become pregnant should avoid both slippery elm and American yellow saffron teas, as they may cause miscarriage.

A most important factor about these herbal teas is that they are not to be taken too close to each other; that is, there should be a lapse of eight to ten hours between taking the slippery elm and the saffron tea.

*Note:* If desired, reverse the order in which saffron tea and slippery elm are taken. In other words, the saffron may be taken in the morning and the slippery elm at night. This may be done to accommodate the work schedule. Remember, they are not to be taken too close to each other, as this would nullify their effects. The slippery elm coats the compromised intestinal wall, helping it to heal, whereas the saffron tea flushes out the liver, the kidneys, and the alimentary canal.

## Ileitis and Psoriasis: A Connecting Link?

It has been brought to my attention that several patients suffering from ileitis (inflammation of the intestines) have shown tendencies toward developing psoriasis. This is especially noted in cases where the ileitis is severe. Doctors connected with research in ileitis feel there is a link between the two diseases, but they have no explanation. In light of what has been presented thus far in this treatise, a possible cause seems to evolve. If the theory I have been working on is correct, a seepage of toxins permeates the intestinal walls and invades the lymph and blood circulatory system. Anything that causes the intestinal walls to break down can, in turn, cause that same seepage to take place, rendering the patient prone to septicemia (toxic buildup in the blood). Psoriasis, or other dermatologic problems, would naturally follow as the body attempts to rid itself of accumulated poisons. Ileitis, especially if severe, most certainly compromises the intestinal walls, thus strengthening what I consider to be a reasonable explanation for connecting the two diseases. Perhaps it would be well for Western researchers to consider using slippery elm in cases of ileitis. The Chinese have used it successfully for centuries.

## Chamomile Tea

Chamomile (*Anthemis nobilis*) tea, one of the oldest and best-known home remedies, grows abundantly almost everywhere. Most health food stores are well supplied with this tea. Chamomile tea may be used as an occasional alternate to saffron, because it is believed that the two herbs work similarly on the body.

Numerous benefits have been attributed to chamomile, including the alleviation of kidney, bronchial, and bladder problems and, when chamomile and bittersweet are combined as an ointment, even bruises and sprains. The most widely recognized use of chamomile by herbalists, however, is as a tonic for the body. It is also one of the most aromatic and pleasant-tasting teas available.

As mentioned earlier, some of my patients with psoriatic lesions on their faces were pleasantly surprised with good results when they steeped saffron and allowed the gentle fumes to rise up, engulfing the face. Using chamomile in the same fashion has also been met with a measure of success. Although chamomile tea is often recommended, saffron tea should be taken more frequently. Chamomile tea should be prepared in the same way as saffron tea. *Caution:* Drinking chamomile tea is not advised if the patient has a ragweed allergy.

## Mullein Tea

Mullein (*Verbascum thapsus*) is the fourth herbal tea specifically suggested for psoriasis. Fresh leaves for the making of tea are preferred, if available. If they are not available, dried leaves will do. The drinking of mullein tea should begin after slippery elm tea has been taken for about ten days.

### Preparation of Mullein Tea

Crumble or crush a teaspoon of mullein leaves and place in a cup. Pour a pint of boiling water over it, and allow it to steep for thirty minutes.

Strain, cool, and drink, not necessarily all at once, but over the course of three or four hours.

Note that in the case of mullein tea, a full teaspoon should be used and the brew should stand for thirty minutes before drinking. It should also be noted that mullein and, in fact, all the dried herbs for making the teas discussed in this chapter should always be stored in the refrigerator. If they aren't, they may become buggy, especially in the summer, even if packaged properly.

# Watermelon Seed Tea

Watermelon (*Citrullus vulgaris*) seed tea has been known for its effectiveness as a diuretic and has been credited with helping remedy bladder infections for centuries. I suggest this tea to my patients as a substitute for saffron, to aid in flushing out the urinary system. Watermelon seed tea is available commercially in the form of loose tea or in tea bags.

## Preparation of Watermelon Seed Tea

Two tablespoons of the tea are boiled for five minutes in a pint of water. This mixture is then covered and allowed to stand until cool before drinking. One cup taken three or four times a day is suggested.

# CHAPTER 8

# The Role of the Spine

T
he role the spine plays in the phenomenon of psoriasis is far more profound than ordinarily assumed. This chapter dealing with the spine and its neural connections may seem a bit technical for the average reader. I hope it will help others, however, especially professionals, to understand why manual adjustments of the spine are an important part of the therapy suggested in the Edgar Cayce works. It is my purpose to answer the questions of both lay and professional readers as simply yet as thoroughly as possible. I hope to encourage active use of spinal adjustments whenever possible by showing that the reasoning behind them is solidly founded on scientific facts.

If it is difficult for you to see the connection between the spinal column and skin diseases, you are not alone. For a long time I did not appreciate their interrelation myself, and neither did most of my chiropractic colleagues and medical friends. However, new consciousness that recognizes the oneness of all things is now emerging. This idea of oneness is really not new; it has been discussed and respected since the days of Paracelsus, Hippocrates, and Pythagoras, but the concept is being rekindled in our present age and is often referred to as "holism." As mentioned earlier, when it is applied to health care, we speak of "holistic medicine." Granted, without a basic understanding of the body's mechanisms, it is next to impossible to appreciate the plausibility of the holistic view of health and disease. Francis Pottenger's *Symptoms of Visceral Disease* states, "Diseases cannot be divided into those of this and that organ; for the human body is a unit. One part cannot be diseased without affecting other parts. No organ can be understood, except in its relationship to other organs and to the body as a whole." These principles are the foundations of the holistic approach to healing.

It is readily understood that the nervous system controls the various functions of the body. If it does not function properly, the whole body, or some part of it, will feel the effects to a greater or lesser degree.

Since our ultimate goal is to get to the root causes of psoriasis and our theory involves the integrity of the walls of the intestinal tract, it behooves us to at least investigate its neural connections, that is, where they originate and what may possibly happen if the normal nerve impulses are altered.

The upper intestinal tract is supplied by nerve impulses emanating from the middorsal vertebrae (the area located between the shoulder blades). If these nerve roots are traumatized by direct injury, curvature of the spine, or *subluxations* (misaligned vertebrae), the normal flow of nerve energy may be disturbed. In fact, one discourse by Cayce clearly states that even one subluxation can cause psoriasis by the effect an impinged nerve or nerves would have on the normal blood circulation to the walls of portions of the intestinal tract. Normal circulation would be impaired, thus causing an impoverishment of these walls, which leads to their eventual breakdown. This, in turn, will render them more permeable to toxic elements. The thinning of the intestinal walls is not only conceivable but predictable. The intestinal walls can become so porous on a microscopic level that seepage of toxic elements can readily find their way into the lymphatics and bloodstream by a process of osmosis. If this "poisoning" is not counteracted, the kidneys and the liver, the major filtering systems of the body, become overtaxed, and the body calls into play its next backup system, the skin, to eliminate the toxins—hence the outward manifestation of psoriasis.

## Your Spine

To study the intricate workings of the spine is to delve into a marvel of living architecture and function. Each vertebra is positioned perfectly in relation to every other, to provide both maximum strength and a flexibility that sometimes, as in the case of dancers, comes close to simulating the movements of a snake. This places the human spine in the category of a biological engineering miracle. Add to this the spine's primary function of protecting the "lifeline" of the body, the spinal cord, and you begin to see the capabilities of a human mechanism that scientists estimate took 100 million years to evolve.

Of the 206 bones in the adult skeleton, 33 comprise the backbone, or spinal column. These thirty-three are known as the vertebrae. In comparison to other bones, the vertebrae are considered small, but their purpose is anything but small. These thirty-three individual, distinct, highly engineered bones are separated into five divisions. The smallest bones are the *cervical (neck) vertebrae,* which allow their division a wider range of motion than the rest of the spine. The *dorsal* (or *thoracic) vertebrae* are twelve in number and make up the upper back; they begin at just below the seventh cervical vertebrae. Heavier than the cervical vertebrae, the dorsals also hold the ribs in place at junctions called *articular facets,* special disk-shaped indentations. The next five vertebrae are located in the lower back. Called the *lumbar vertebrae,* they bear most of the body's weight. The position of each facet on each vertebra, relative to the next, plays a major role in what is termed a *vertebral subluxation* or *vertebral lesion.*

There are four distinct curves in the adult spine. At birth, however, there is only one continuous curve, a generalized convex, or *kyphotic,* curve. After birth, as the child begins to develop and bend his or her neck, the cervical curve, which is concave, or *lordotic,* begins to appear. A similar process occurs in the lower back, forming the concave curve of the lumbar spine. The four distinct spinal curves are featured in the illustration on page 122. Note that I have specifically pointed out the sixth and seventh dorsal (thoracic), third cervical, ninth dorsal, and fourth lumbar vertebrae. These are the vertebral segments that, due to their neural connections, are directly involved in combating psoriasis.

Beneath the lumbar vertebrae is the *sacrum,* which, at birth, is really five separate smaller vertebrae that finally fuse at about age twenty-five to form a wedge-shaped bone, which fits between the two hip bones. Beneath the sacrum, at the very end of the spine, is the *coccyx,* known as the tailbone. This, too, begins as separate small bones (four in number), which fuse into one structure in the adult.

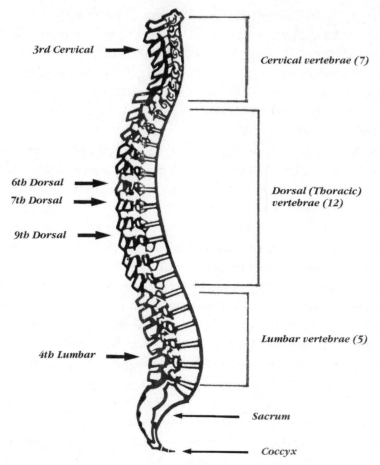

3rd Cervical ➤

Cervical vertebrae (7)

6th Dorsal ➤
7th Dorsal ➤

9th Dorsal ➤

Dorsal (Thoracic)
vertebrae (12)

Lumbar vertebrae (5)

4th Lumbar ➤

Sacrum ◄

Coccyx ◄

The spine.

Between each of the cervical, thoracic, and lumbar vertebrae, and
between the fifth lumbar and the sacrum, are specialized cushions,
the *intervertebral disks.* These disks, which make up about 25 percent
of the adult's spine length, are designed to absorb shock and keep the
bones from grinding against one another. They also permit greater
flexibility between the vertebrae and allow for changes in body balance. Being relatively soft and flexible, they easily adapt to changes
in posture. By separating one vertebra from another, the disks also
provide openings that allow the nerves that emerge from the spinal

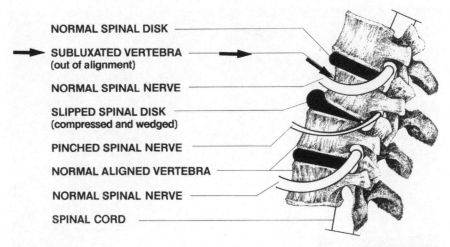

NORMAL SPINAL DISK

SUBLUXATED VERTEBRA
(out of alignment)

NORMAL SPINAL NERVE

SLIPPED SPINAL DISK
(compressed and wedged)

PINCHED SPINAL NERVE

NORMAL ALIGNED VERTEBRA

NORMAL SPINAL NERVE

SPINAL CORD

Spinal subluxation.

cord to pass, unobstructed, between the vertebrae. The openings, the *intervertebral foramina,* can be altered in size and shape to an abnormal degree by injury, poor posture, spinal defects, or idiopathic (unknown) causes.

Such changes in one of the openings can cause a pressure point and/ or an inflammation of nerve roots located at that opening. The chiropractic theory of health and disease holds that this condition, referred to as a subluxation, is a major cause of abnormal states in the body that can result in a wide range of symptoms, from pain to abnormal physiological function. Osteopaths use the term *spinal lesion* to describe essentially the same thing. The treatment in both professions is also basically the same: spinal adjustment or manipulation (an ancient art) to eliminate the pressure point.

To go into a detailed anatomical discussion about the neural connections between the spinal cord and the intestinal tract would serve no useful purpose here. It is enough to simply state that the nerve supply to the upper intestinal tract, in particular to the areas of the *duodenal-jejunal junction* (*flexure*), originate in the middorsal area of the spine, the sixth and seventh dorsals being the principal vertebrae involved.

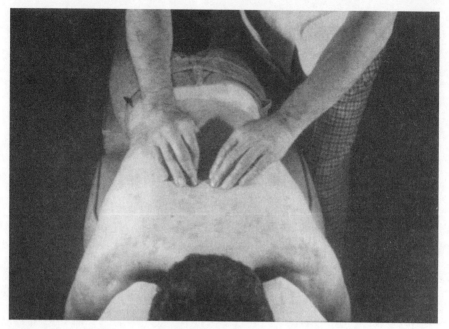

Palpation of the sixth and seventh dorsal vertebrae.

## Innervation of the Skin

Can spinal adjustments conceivably aid the skin *directly* as well as revitalizing the internal organs that eliminate waste and neutralize toxins? I contend that they can and do—particularly general, full-spine adjustments.

The skin is an organ. It is, in fact, the largest organ of the body. Every cell in every organ of the human body must receive electrical (nerve) energy to remain in a state of health, and this organ is no exception. There is, indeed, a nerve supply to the skin itself, and, as Pottenger states, "The structures of the skin, as far as physiologists have been able to determine, possess only sympathetic nerves receiving innervation from the thoracic (dorsal) and upper three lumbar segments."

Therefore, from the first dorsal down to the third lumbar, a total of fifteen vertebral segments, there is a relationship between the spine and the structures of the skin by way of the nerves that emanate from between these vertebrae. Due to this anatomical-physiological fact, spinal adjustments can indeed benefit dermal structures, whether or not a skin disease is actually present.

## Contradictions?

Several questions will probably occur to you regarding what I have said so far. The following premises, discussed at length in the preceding chapters, may seem contradictory: first, that psoriasis is caused by a thinning of the upper intestinal walls; second, that it is due to chronic constipation; third, that poor diet is to blame; and now, that the spine is out of alignment. Can all these statements be equally valid? Is there any one cause that is common to all cases?

It should be understood that these different causes of psoriasis can work in conjunction with one another. The *only* apparent common denominator among psoriatics is that, for one reason or another, the patient's body cannot handle the toxic buildup within it. The organs that normally eliminate toxins fail to do the job effectively, and so the skin, the body's secondary line of defense, is pressed into service. If we consider psoriasis a condition rather than a specific disease, we will stop looking for *the* cause and seriously examine the *causes.* It is up to the treating physician to determine why the patient builds up toxins. When the physician solves that riddle, he or she can proceed intelligently in recommending therapy. More often than not, good results will follow, given adequate time.

## The Spinal Adjustment: Rationale and Technique

When people consider having a spinal adjustment administered by a competent chiropractor or osteopath, it is usually because they have pain in some area of the spine. This is well and good because, in the vast majority of such cases, an adjustment is just what is needed and will most likely clear up the problem if misaligned vertebrae are the basic cause.

Rarely, however, do people realize that a spinal adjustment may be needed in connection with the function of specific organs, particularly those of the abdominal viscera, because there is often no telltale sign of pain when one or more of these organs is not functioning properly. To be sure, there may be other signs, such as jaundice, malaise, or headache, but people do not readily connect these symptoms with the spine. I believe this is one reason some patients cannot appreciate the benefits of spinal adjustments in relation to psoriasis. They are more familiar with the chiropractor's or osteopath's role in treating pain than with his or her role in making spinal adjustments to release nerve energy needed for proper functioning of the abdominal organs. A quick reference to accepted textbooks on anatomy and physiology will confirm the wisdom that spinal adjustments can play a *major* role in psoriasis therapy. The beneficial effect they may have on the digestive tract, the alimentary canal, the glandular centers, and the skin itself warrants serious consideration.

Trying to prove whether a subluxation is present may end in frustration, for in many cases, it cannot be demonstrated clinically. It can, however, be assumed. Whether a patient responds favorably is all that really matters and, quite frankly, all that the patient cares about. J. E. Bourdillon, the past president of the North American Academy of Manipulative Medicine and a former consultant orthopedic surgeon to the Gloucestershire Royal Hospital in England, effectively reminds us in his book *Spinal Manipulation* that practical results, rather than scientific analysis, have always been the main aim of physicians. Our modern preoccupation with science makes us too easily forget that "[o]nly a few generations ago medicine was an art, and the large majority of medical and surgical treatment was based on the results of practical experience rather than on firm scientific foundation."

Why is the spinal adjustment so vital to the psoriatic? Because not only can it help restore the normal integrity of the intestinal wall that is essential to an alleviation of the condition, but it can also make possible the one thing a psoriatic is most interested in: a *permanent cure.* If the entire psoriatic syndrome has its *origin* in spinal subluxations, correcting these subluxations should be the first line of attack against the disease. It is my conclusion, therefore, according to logic and theory, that if one has the required adjustments of the spine and follows through with all the other measures called for in the regimen, a permanent cure is possible.

Only time and further research can provide the final answer regarding permanence of the cure. One thing is certain in following this alternative approach: if it is successful, the patient knows that he or she is then permanently in control of the condition.

## Spinal Manipulation and Stimulation

The spinal adjustment (adjustment of the vertebrae) goes back to the days of the Egyptians. The modern resurgence of this age-old form of therapy began in 1895, when D. D. Palmer of Davenport, Iowa, literally "adjusted" the vertebrae of a man named Harvey Lillard and, in performing that manipulation, cured him of deafness he had suffered following a fall eighteen years earlier. That incident launched the present-day chiropractic movement.

Some people resist chiropractic adjustment merely because of the sounds that occur when an adjustment is taking place. It sounds like the doctor is cracking bones, although he or she is doing no such thing. The cracking sound is created by the vacuum release that occurs when two vertebrae are slightly moved, thus reducing the subluxation that may be present.

The primary areas of the spine to be adjusted and/or stimulated are illustrated below.

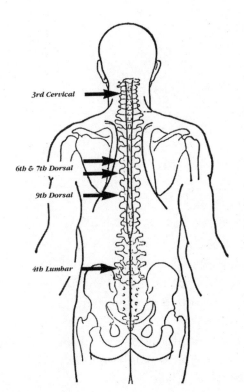

Adjustments of the spine.

Even those who do not like being adjusted invariably enjoy stimulation of the spinal segments by manual massage and/or the use of various modalities. The modalities I speak of are primarily three: electrical stimulation administered by a doctor or a trained assistant, use of the Morfam Master Massager, and the Oster Hand Massager. In some cases, these units may take the place of spinal adjustments and prove to be quite effective, or they may be used in conjunction with spinal adjustments. The object of these units is to stimulate the nerve roots as they emanate from between the vertebrae (particularly the sixth and the seventh dorsal) and surrounding tissue.

These units (except for the electrical stimulator) are readily available to the general public. There are many brands of massagers, some better than others. Look at as many as you can, and if one is approved by your medical doctor, have it at home to use at your discretion. It is a safe way to activate the spine and stimulate the nerves, and it simply feels good!

In recent years, the "activator" method of adjusting spinal subluxations has steadily grown in popularity with both trained chiropractors and their patients. A specially designed mechanical device is used manually to reduce or remove subluxations. It has proven to be quite effective in many cases and is easy on the patient.

A spinal subluxation does not have to be extensive or even discernible on X-rays to be present. It can be as minute as a fraction of a millimeter yet cause excruciating pain. Conversely, the slightest adjustment (a tiny "click," if you will) can offer symptomatic relief, thus the growing popularity of the activator method of adjusting. Only a slight corrective movement administered by the chiropractor with the activator device can offer incredible relief. I can recall my anatomy professor in college saying to us that a spinal deviation (subluxation) no greater than the thickness of a piece of paper can cause an inflammatory reaction at the site that results in crippling pain. The good news is that the slightest corrective adjustment can offer relief.

To summarize, manipulation or stimulation of the spine helps maintain the all-important coordinating function of the nervous system. It is therefore conceivable that a person suffering from psoriasis can benefit from spinal manipulations by virtue of the fact that the intestinal tract, as well as the structure of the skin itself, is supplied by nerve impulses emanating from the dorsal spine. As Hippocrates said, "Look well to the spine for the cause of disease."

# CHAPTER 9

# External Applications

The most important thing to grasp about external (topical) applications is that *all* of them are merely palliative. As effective as some of them are in soothing the inflamed skin of psoriasis, they do not get to the root cause of the disease. The oils and ointments make the skin more pliable, rendering it less prone to splitting and cracking, which is a major problem for many psoriasis sufferers. Removal of scales and less new scaling seem to be a fringe benefit of using these creams and oils. Personally, I believe they aid in healing the surface cells by acting therapeutically on the lesions as if they were wounds.

No one can deny that both the sun and ultraviolet-light treatments have often helped alleviate surface lesions and have kept some sufferers clear for several months. An equal number, however, have experienced the pain and discouragement of the return of their lesions, often worse than before. The obvious reason for their return is that the root cause of the disease is not affected by surface applications.

The following measures are suggested for the purpose of soothing the surface areas and alleviating at least some of the distressing symptoms, particularly itching. Although they will not address the root cause of the condition, they can offer comfort while the basic internal cause is being corrected. By trial and error, my patients choose those that work best for them. I mention only those that are easily applied and readily available.

- An olive oil–peanut oil mixture
- Castor oil
- Cuticura soap, ointment, and shampoo
- Resinol
- Vaseline (white) and the new Vaseline cocoa butter, Baker's P&S Liquid, Ray's Ointment (for the hairline)
- Vitamin E
- Epsom or Dead Sea salts baths
- Fume and/or steam baths, wet sauna
- Sunlight and ultraviolet light
- Sodium bicarbonate (baking soda) baths and Aveeno baths
- Witch hazel, Listerine, Glyco-Thymoline sitz bath for the genital area
- Electrical stimulation and ultrasound (professionally applied)
- Olive oil–tincture of myrrh massage
- Hydrophilic ointment
- Physiotherapy at home
- Pure, organic coconut oil

## Olive Oil–Peanut Oil Mixture

A mixture of equal parts olive oil and peanut oil is one of the most soothing applications. (Peanut oil is not to be used externally if there is an allergy to peanuts.) It can be massaged into individual lesions or over the entire body, and it helps prevent the cracking of dried lesions. This mixture is most useful in the winter, when the humidity indoors is low due to artificial heat. It is also the best application for the scalp when a viselike feeling grips the head, and lesions characterized by a white, snow-capped appearance as well as lumps are seen or felt all over the scalp.

I suggest the use of the olive oil–peanut oil mixture more than any other external oil application at home because, as mentioned, it helps heal the surface cells, enhances the skin's pliability, and is relatively easy to clean when applied to the scalp. This technique is detailed in chapter 12.

If the lesions are thick and disfiguring throughout the torso, I advise my patients to massage the mixture well into the lesions and then place a plastic bag, such as those used by dry cleaners, over the torso. Openings are cut for the head and the arms, and the bag is cut to waist length and then worn underneath pajamas. In the morning, the plastic bag is removed and discarded. Plastic bags can be used on the thighs or the legs as well, but not at the same time as on the torso. There must be enough body surface exposed to the air for the skin to breathe efficiently. Under *no* circumstances should plastic bags or plastic wrap be used on children, since this may accidentally cause strangulation or suffocation.

Two or three bag treatments a week are usually sufficient, even in the most severe cases. Naturally, as the condition improves, this type of application can be cut down until it is no longer necessary. A similar application may be used for the arms, particularly the elbows; the only difference being that plastic wrap is used instead of the bags to seal off the skin. I have found this method to be a good substitute for the more elaborate occlusion suits used by some psoriatics. The plastic bags or wrap are simply discarded after use and cost very little.

Some patients have problems using plastic wrap or bags directly on the skin. They find it hot, sweaty, and generally uncomfortable. Instead they wear white cotton gloves or socks on the hands or feet after massaging them with the olive oil–peanut oil mixture or castor oil. For large areas such as the back, the chest, or the abdomen, they rub the oils in deeply, allow them to be absorbed for a few minutes, then put on a white cotton overshirt or sweatshirt and retire for the night. Frankly, I prefer this to the age-old method of using plastic or rubber wrapping directly over the oil. For one thing, it is much more comfortable. Cloth also allows the skin to breathe and is less restrictive. The difference, however, is obvious; cotton garments are not disposable. Laundering the garments after use must be made part of the routine. Many patients feel that the advantages of using white cotton garments, without the plastic wrap, far outweigh the inconvenience of laundering. White cotton also does not contain dyes characteristic of color clothing that may irritate the skin.

A good tip when washing the oil-stained clothing is to add a cup of sodium bicarbonate (baking soda) to the water during the wash cycle to help remove the oil. Needless to say the wash load should contain only the clothes used for this purpose, even if it means accumulating them in their own hamper for a few days before laundering. Realize that there will always be a certain amount of staining of the clothing or linens, no matter how carefully they are washed, so patients should not use their best garments or linens for this purpose.

The only drawback in applying the olive oil–peanut oil mixture is that you may smell a bit like a salad! Although I prefer the unscented version, there is on the market an olive oil–peanut oil mixture with a lovely almond scent that makes all the difference. It is available through Baar Products and the Heritage Store (see appendix D).

## Castor Oil

Castor oil has more benefits than most people realize. Not only is it a natural cathartic when taken internally, but castor oil is a most effective topical application for several conditions not typically associated with its use. I have successfully used it on warts and sprains and strains in athletic injuries, and even on myself when I had a kidney stone attack.

In psoriasis cases, castor oil should be viewed as a topical application to be used particularly on heavy, circumscribed lesions. (See the case of J.R. in the photo section.) The castor oil should be "cold-pressed, AA-USP," which is available through Baar Products and the Heritage Store. The best use of the oil is to gently rub a liberal amount into the lesions and leave it on overnight or at least for several hours. Because of its viscosity (thickness), it is not used as a scalp treatment or for massaging the body in general, as it would be rather difficult to remove. On smaller, circumscribed areas, however, it can be most effective.

There are certain combinations that increase the usefulness of the oil. Castor oil rubbed into a lesion, followed immediately by Resinol applied right over the oil, helps relieve itching of the lesion. Rubbing a paste made from castor oil combined with sodium bicarbonate (baking soda) into thick, scaly heels or other heavily encrusted lesions has shown remarkable results in most patients. If the skin is cracked, however, this combination may prove to be somewhat caustic and should not be used until the skin has healed over. In such cases, the olive oil–peanut oil mixture or plain castor oil, without the baking soda, is used instead. Other soothing applications are Vaseline cocoa butter and/or coconut oil.

## Cuticura Soap, Ointment, and Shampoo

Cuticura soap, ointment, and shampoo are among the oldest bath products available. This soap is widely used in cases of psoriasis when following my regimen. As mentioned earlier, the only time it is not used is if the sufferer has an allergic reaction to one of its ingredients, which is rarely the case. Cuticura ointment has been very effective on large patches of psoriasis, particularly common vulgaris, which are well circumscribed and raised above the surface of the skin (acanthosis). It can be used alone or in combination with castor oil. A plastic wrapping over the lesion is needed to prevent soiling of clothing or linens, as this compound is capable of heavy staining and discoloration. Mr. William Culmone, whose case is described in chapter 2, used Cuticura ointment, combined with castor oil, extensively, with excellent results. Cuticura shampoo is often effective on the scalp but may have to be ordered from a local druggist or through Baar Products.

## Resinol

Resinol is recommended to prevent itching. As mentioned earlier, I have found it quite helpful in combination with castor oil in the event that Cuticura ointment is unavailable. Many anti-itch products are on the market these days, and I advise people to use whatever seems to help.

## Vaseline, Baker's P&S Liquid, and Ray's Ointment

Three products that can be used along the hairline, on small, circumscribed lesions of the scalp, and behind the ears are Vaseline, Baker's P&S Liquid, and Ray's Ointment. Although quite different in their makeup, they all have repeatedly proven to be helpful when used in these areas.

## Using Vitamin E

Although vitamin E was not mentioned earlier relative to psoriasis, one patient tried rubbing it into heavily scaled areas, using the liquid and/or cream form, and achieved encouraging results.

The patient explained that Cuticura ointment did loosen the scales but that the vitamin E did not need to be worked in so vigorously. It removed the scales more quickly, and the lesions broke up faster. She used only the vitamin E cream (5,000 IU) and no longer had to apply the oils and ointment before going to sleep at night. This substance tends to prevent thickening of the lesions, is easy to apply, is relatively inexpensive, and has little odor. Another advantage is that it also keeps the skin soft throughout the day. Similar results have often occurred using hydrophilic ointment.

## Epsom and Dead Sea Salts Baths

An Epsom salts bath is one of the most beneficial, cleansing procedures readily available to most patients. The water should be comfortably hot and the tub filled enough so the patient's entire body, up to the neck, can be immersed. The water should contain about four pounds of Epsom salts. To use only a cup or two would not be very effective in most cases of psoriasis. In the case of Dead Sea salts, a cup and a half is all that is necessary in a tub of comfortably hot water.

I advise remaining in the tub for about twenty or thirty minutes and reheating the water periodically as it cools. It is best to keep the water temperature between 106 and 108 degrees Fahrenheit, but keep it at what feels comfortable to you. If possible, these baths should be taken at least twice a week, followed with a good olive oil–peanut oil massage before retiring for the night.

There are precautions, however, that must be observed. Epsom salts baths *should not* be taken if:

- There is a heart or blood-pressure problem.
- The skin is cracked or is so sensitive that the salts cause a painful burning sensation.
- The person is alone (in case of dizziness or faintness).
- There is no one available to help a person into or out of the tub should he or she be geriatric or severely arthritic.

The key word is *caution.* Be sensible; don't be in a hurry. An Epsom salts bath should be one of the most soothing, gentle cleansing procedures experienced by the psoriatic. My patients make it so when I insist that they take the necessary precautions.

## Fume and/or Steam Baths and Wet Sauna

This subject has been adequately covered in chapter 5. It is listed here because it may also be classified as an external application. In essence, the fume or steam bath may be thought of as an external application that aids internal cleansing. Therefore, I feel it is fitting to mention this procedure in both chapters.

## Sunlight and Ultraviolet Light

Natural sunlight is the best form of ultraviolet light for the psoriatic, but with two stipulations: never be exposed to the point of getting sunburned, and never sunbathe between the hours of 11:00 A.M. and 3:00 P.M. These precautions apply to everyone, psoriatic or not, when you take into account the warnings astronomers have issued in recent years about increased sunspot activity and the alarming destruction of our Earth's protective ozone layer. More sunspot activity means more radioactive light coming into our atmosphere, leading to a higher incidence of skin cancer. So don't attempt to soak up too many rays in one sitting, even outside the midday hours.

Since some people are more sensitive to the sun's rays than others are, we cannot say exactly how much is too much. Ten minutes could have little effect on one person and scald another. If a sunscreen is used in a lotion, it should have an SPF of at least 15 and be placed on areas that have no lesions. There is also a decided difference between ten minutes in the sun on northern beaches, such as those of the North Atlantic seaboard, and ten minutes in the tropical sun, such as in the Caribbean. Gradual exposure is the safest way. Only time and experience can tell you what is right for you, but if it is a question of coming out of the sun sooner or later, make it sooner.

If the skin does become burned, I advise the application of Glyco-Thymoline, apple cider vinegar diluted in water, or any of the known sunburn lotions that have proven to be helpful. Although apple cider vinegar diluted in water has been used successfully, I would not use it on open lesions. On areas where there are no lesions, it may prove to be a godsend. It is best to try it on small areas first and observe the reaction. As always, caution is advised, as some individuals may react unfavorably.

The most important thing is to exercise common sense. People particularly sensitive to the sun should avoid exposing their skin to it. However, ultraviolet light from the sun can still benefit psoriatics if they wear lightweight clothing. Even if patients are not especially sensitive to the sun, they should be careful not to overexpose themselves and should choose carefully the hours of the day to sunbathe. In general, swimming in clean salt water followed by moderate exposure to the sun is, in my opinion, the most beneficial external treatment available to the psoriatic.

## Artificial Ultraviolet Light

Surprisingly, the external application of ultraviolet light has played a relatively minor role in the clearing of my patients' psoriasis. For those who had an ultraviolet light home unit, I did not discourage its use as long as it was prescribed by a dermatologist who gave proper instructions. Even under these conditions there can be dangers. On several occasions, the overuse of a patient's home unit caused a most severe reaction, marked by swollen eyelids, hypersensitive skin, and swollen lips, which took several days to overcome.

Although tanning salons continue to gain in popularity throughout the United States, the dangers involved should be clearly recognized. The American Medical Association (AMA) warned against the use of cosmetic tanning as reported in a June 17, 1985, Associated Press article titled "AMA Cautions against Tanning." The article stated that the position of the AMA was that

> there is no known medical benefit from cosmetic tanning. . . .
> The AMA's science council cited a recent study concluding that high-intensity, ultraviolet radiation emitted by even the newest and safest devices, has no known beneficial effects to human health and is potentially dangerous. It said short-term and long-term exposure can cause changes in the skin, compromising its ability to ward off disease, causing it to degenerate and making it more likely to produce tumors.

Psoriatics and anyone else influenced by the public craze for tanning should take heed of these warnings.

## Sodium Bicarbonate (Baking Soda) and Aveeno Baths

General itching, or pruritus, is one of the most irritating problems the psoriatic has to face, especially during the early stages of therapy. The one thing a patient must never do is scratch! The result will only be increased irritation, bleeding, possible infection, and the formation of new psoriatic lesions.

In many cases, about one pound of baking soda in a tub of comfortably hot water is very effective in relieving the itch. At times, I recommend two pounds in a tub of water. It may not work in every case, but it is inexpensive and certainly worth a try. Another product is Aveeno, which has an oatmeal base and is added to the tub of water. Results have been generally encouraging. This product is available in any drugstore. The idea is to find what works best for each patient and use it. A paste of sodium bicarbonate and apple cider vinegar often relieves the itch in circumscribed areas.

It is most interesting that at least one patient called to inform me of his almost immediate relief of generalized itching when he put one teaspoon of sodium bicarbonate in a glass of water and drank it. Within a few minutes after he drank the water, the itch that was torturing him subsided. Undoubtedly, a shift in the chemistry of his body took place, the sodium bicarbonate rendering it more alkaline, or at least neutralizing the acidity throughout his system. Whatever the reason, the procedure was harmless but highly effective and may be helpful in some patients when generalized itching occurs.

## Witch Hazel, Listerine, and Glyco-Thymoline

Witch hazel is a useful addition to the fume bath for psoriatics, as mentioned earlier: a tablespoon of witch hazel is placed in half a pint of water, which is used in the steam cabinet. In addition to helping to remove toxins, witch hazel placed in the water of a fume bath provides another benefit—relief from itching. Sometimes, when all else fails, applying it directly to the irritated area proves helpful. It is applied with a cotton ball, or if there are no open cracks in the skin, the witch hazel can be applied directly with the fingers or the palm of the hand.

Listerine, the popular throat antiseptic, is used primarily on areas of the scalp when itching is a problem. It is used by simply dabbing it on small lesions or diluting in warm water (about 20 percent Listerine to 80 percent water, making one quart) and using it as a general rinse following a shampoo.

Glyco-Thymoline is a red, alkaline mouthwash that has been on the market for many years. It may be ordered from a local druggist or from the suppliers listed in appendix D. It, too, is applied directly to the skin to relieve itching or sunburn or is diluted and used as a final rinse after a shampoo. Glyco-Thymoline has also been suggested as an alkalizer and intestinal antiseptic when taken internally. Most patients take just four or five drops in a glass of water before bedtime. It has been described in the Cayce material as an alimentary canal purifier, most desirable to the psoriatic, especially for those suffering from psoriatic arthritis. Patients usually take it five nights out of the week.

## Psoriasis or Eczema of the Genital Area

Psoriatic lesions and/or the rash of eczema on the genitals are probably the most irritating, uncomfortable, and tormenting annoyance a person can experience. We have found the use of a small sitz bath using Glyco-Thymoline or Lavoris (both mouthwashes) most helpful as an external application. Depending on the size of the person, a small basin of lukewarm water, about three-quarters full, is placed in an empty bathtub. About a cup of Glyco-Thymoline or Lavoris is added to the water. One then squats down in the basin, soaking the entire genital area for about ten or fifteen minutes. (Geriatric patients may need help with this.) Then the patient stands and pats the area dry, without rinsing. About fifteen to twenty minutes later, the patient may shower. (Glyco-Thymoline may be ordered from the product suppliers listed in appendix D; Lavoris is readily available in most drugstores.)

# Electrical Stimulation and Ultrasound

The electrical stimulation I refer to here comes from a physiotherapy unit, a muscle stimulator, which is applied only by a physician to the primary areas of the spine directly involved in psoriasis, namely, the third cervical; the sixth, seventh, and ninth dorsal; and the fourth lumbar vertebrae (see chapter 8).

By applying small electrical pads to these specific areas, impulses may stimulate the nerve roots emanating from between these vertebrae, helping to ensure nerve flow to the glandular and internal organs that are involved. It is gentle in application, relaxing, and generally may help the overall picture. This therapy, along with spinal adjustments and deep massage along the spine, is the best natural method I know of that can help ensure normal nerve flow to the internal organs as well as the skin itself.

Studies conducted at Stanford University show that using ultrasound to heat the body (controlled hyperthermia) helps clear the skin of psoriasis. This form of treatment is based simply on evidence that heat appears to benefit psoriasis sufferers, as psoriasis generally improves in the summer and gets worse in the winter. This therapy seems to work best on small, confined lesions.

I use ultrasound primarily in cases involving psoriasis of the palms. At times, the skin of the palms can become so thick with scales, stiffness, and cracking that it resembles elephant skin. The ultrasound, used with the patient's hands submerged in a basin of warm water, helps soften the heavily callused palms, allowing subsequent oil/electric mitt home treatment to be more effective (see chapter 13). This type of therapy should also be administered only by a physician or a trained physician's assistant. It is mentioned here only for the benefit of those doctors who have access to an ultrasound unit but may not be aware of its effectiveness in such cases. Vaseline cocoa butter massaged into the hands, which are then placed into white gym socks and left overnight, is also very helpful.

## Olive Oil–Tincture of Myrrh Massage

A thorough massage of the abdomen using a mixture of equal parts olive oil (heated) and tincture of myrrh may be one of the most beneficial measures a psoriatic patient can take. Concentrated kneading should take place, particularly along the right side of the abdomen. This is the area where congestion of fecal matter is most likely to occur. The action should be directed from below, upward along the right side to the lower right border of the rib cage, then left (slowly) across the stomach area to the left border of the abdomen, then down (slowly) along the left side to the pubic area. This action follows the normal path of the colon and will help move toxic accumulations out of the alimentary canal. If this is done thoroughly, a weekly massage may be all that is necessary. Massaging slowly from right to left in a circular motion not only encourages peristaltic action of the colon, but it also helps stimulate circulation to the upper intestinal tract, the site of the thinning walls.

When my patients have no one available to give them the massage, I show them how to do it themselves. Lying on their back, knees up (to relax the abdomen), they follow the pattern described above. If a sluggish bowel is part of the problem, this type of massage will undoubtedly benefit the patient by enhancing his bowel movements.

## Hydrophilic Ointment

In addition to the topical applications I already mentioned, hydrophilic ointment must be included in the list of creams that I have found to be quite consistent in soothing circumscribed lesions. It is simply rubbed into the lesion, as is the Cuticura ointment, and there is no problem of staining. It must not be used near the eyes and, of course, should be applied only externally. It is a nonprescription item and may be obtained or ordered in any drugstore. I recommend my patients use the non–U.S. pharmacy (USP) type, which is soft and creamy (labeled "Differs from USP"). I found this ointment to be quite effective on open lesions but not on the flexural type of psoriasis, which occurs where skin surfaces meet, such as in the underarms, breast folds, and gluteal (buttocks) crease. The ointment seems to irritate these areas because there is no air space. It is most important to keep these areas dry; in some cases, I have found Johnson's cornstarch-based or talc-based baby powder to be effective.

The hydrophilic ointment, if hardened, can be made more spreadable by combining a full jar of it with half a jar of water in a mixing bowl and whipping with an electric mixer on high speed until the mixture has the consistency of shaving cream. This mixture can then be stored in one large container, or it can be divided into smaller jars.

In this form, the ointment can be used on large areas of the body and will more easily hold moisture. If the soft, creamy type is purchased, mixing is not necessary.

## It Pays to Be Patient

At first glance, all of these applications and procedures may seem to be a lot of bother and difficult to remember. Actually, they are not. Once the ingredients are at my patient's fingertips and the measures are understood, the applications are quite simple to perform—with one additional benefit: the patient can do them at home at his or her own pace. It beats traveling to a psoriatic center perhaps three or four times a week and probably some distance from home. The cost of these items is minimal, and the possible side effects are practically nonexistent. After a while, most people find they do not need all of these measures and can select the ones that best suit their particular condition and circumstances.

It is my contention that external applications help rid the body of lesions because the emulsions, especially the heavier salves, seal off the surface avenues of escape for the toxins. I have observed that these emulsions will work with any ingredients that can safely seal off the lesions. Circumscribed lesions often disappear equally well after applying substances that are completely foreign to one another in their chemical composition. It is well known, for instance, that surface tar derivatives are very helpful, but so are castor oil, olive and peanut oils, vitamin E cream, and vitamin D cream. To this list of "sealants," one could even add adhesive tape! The fact is, they all work to some degree. Some preparations are more pleasant to use and have fewer side effects or inconveniences than others do. It is mainly for these reasons that individuals will find one preferable to another.

It is important to remember when using these applications, that the internal toxins have to get out somehow, and unless the normal channels of elimination have been opened up, new routes of escape will develop through other areas of the skin. (Holding firm to the theory that the toxins are finding their way out through the sweat glands implies that the lesions form because of this toxic exodus.)

It is for this reason that holistic treatment, in which all areas and functions of the body are taken into account, is crucial. Proper elimination of wastes is primary, followed by a diet that is both cleansing and nutritious. The soothing external salves and ointments will cause the toxins to eventually retract and be removed by the now better-functioning excretory system, thus helping to prevent further spreading of the disease.

## Physiotherapy at Home

I have often been asked, especially by conscientious patients, if any physiotherapy units may be used effectively at home. Several kinds are indeed available, and they can be quite helpful.

The five that I consider most important are:

1. Whirlpool—either built in, such as a hot tub, or portable, such as a unit that may be attached to the side of the tub or laid flat in the tub, producing air bubbles. Smaller, self-contained units are available for hands and feet.

2. Steam bath cabinet (for home use)—made of fiberglass with stainless steel and aluminum fittings. The patient sits comfortably in the unit and closes a door, but the head is always exposed. (*Note:* The same precautions apply in using a whirlpool or a home steam cabinet as they do for taking an Epsom salts bath or a professional steam bath.) This is not to be used if the patient has a heart problem.

3. Electrical heat cap, mitts, and boots—used for treatments of the scalp, hands, and feet, respectively, in conjunction with various oils.

4. Humidifier—particularly for use in the winter months, to offset the dry air caused by artificial heating. A humidifier can be very effective in preventing or alleviating winter itch (asteatotic dermatitis). (*Caution:* Units must be thoroughly cleaned out regularly, as spores may form that may be inhaled, causing serious respiratory ailments.)

5. Ultraviolet lamp (optional)—used as directed by the patient's dermatologist.

In addition, every psoriatic should have a juicer and a blender for making fresh vegetable and fruit juices, and a home enema device, especially if constipation is a problem. Never retire for the night without having at least one bowel movement that day.

The above units are readily available to the general public at a nominal cost. In remote areas where professional services are not available, these home units can be a godsend, provided they are used properly and with discretion. They are all a patient needs, from a physiotherapeutic point of view. Again, these products become more worthy of consideration when the convenience of using them in the privacy of one's own home is taken into account.

## The Effect of Wearing Synthetic Fabrics

As mentioned in the previous chapter on eczema, patients who wear nylon or synthetic undergarments sometimes have an adverse reaction to this fabric, especially after their skin has been cleared up. One patient, after doing exceptionally well, came back with her entire torso inflamed. It looked as though the healing process had reversed itself. Upon close inspection and questioning, however, we discovered a perfect outline on her body that followed the contour of her bathing suit. Just prior to this flare-up, the patient had worn a nylon bathing suit. This reaction had been observed before, when another patient wore nylon or synthetic leotards. The line of demarcation could easily be noted. Because skin cannot breathe properly under synthetics, I concluded that these fabrics in fact caused this adverse reaction. Consequently, my advice was to wear only cotton undergarments and bathing suits containing as little synthetic fiber as possible, preferably consisting mainly of cotton. Since I made this observation, my suggestion proved to be beneficial to this patient as well as to several others.

In addition to these, a cool shower or an ice cube placed on a small area may provide relief. There are a number of prescription as well as over-the-counter items available that claim to relieve itching. Whatever works, works! The above nonprescription items are all I ever recommend. Remember, once the internal cleansing process begins to take effect, the annoying itch is the first symptom to disappear, and that is the first sign that the process is working.

## No Substitute for Time

There is one basic thing I insist my patients always keep in mind, especially since this regimen is not a get-well-quick procedure. If I sound redundant, it is my intention to be so. Psoriasis will not disappear until the basic cause has been removed. Since the basic cause is a buildup of internal toxins that has accumulated over an extended period of time, the removal of these toxins is not an overnight process. In following this regimen, it is absolutely essential to *give time a chance.* Without it, the effort is worthless. Discipline is an absolute must if results are to be expected, and this regimen may not be as rigorous as one might imagine.

One of my patients summed up the attitude needed to apply the psoriasis regimen with complete success in these simple, wise words: "It is a discipline only until it becomes a habit—then it takes over!"

# CHAPTER 10

# Right Thinking: The Role of the Mind

Albert Schweitzer was once asked the question "What's wrong with men today?" His answer, sharp and to the point, was, "Men simply don't think!" Of course, not all men fall into that category, but this in itself raises another question. Of those people who *do* "think," what are they thinking about? Are their thoughts of a constructive nature or are they destructive? You see, the nature of their thoughts builds the world around them. Their bodies and circumstances, whether or not they believe it, are the end result of the thoughts they harbor within.

The philosopher James Allen, in his classic work *As a Man Thinketh,* said, "Of all the beautiful truths pertaining to the soul, none is more gladdening or fruitful of divine promise and confidence than this; that man is the master of thought, the molder of character, and the maker and shaper of condition, environment, and destiny."

Once a person realizes that, to a great extent, he has the power to *choose* his thoughts, he would be foolish if he did not decide on a constructive course of thinking. If he then holds to it with faith in the creative power of thought, he will eventually benefit and improve all areas of his life. He is free to choose.

What must we do to realize the healthy life, the good life, the life worth living? We must exercise "right thinking." Right thinking means choosing a pattern of thoughts designed to benefit a person without bringing harm to others. Sometimes subtle changes in our thoughts bring about incredible results. For instance, normally no one wants to be sick. But if you say or think the words "I don't want to be sick," you focus your thinking on sickness, and chances are you will draw sickness to yourself. For as you think, so shall you become. The difference in right thinking is not to say to yourself, "I don't want to be sick," which is a negative statement, but "I am healthy!" which makes a positive, constructive *present-tense* declaration. If this affirmation is repeated often enough, it will eventually enter your subconscious mind and manifest itself outwardly in your life. This will be discussed later in this chapter, in the section titled "The Mental Formula of Émile Coué."

## The Wisdom of Thomas Troward

Thomas Troward was one of the world's leading exponents on the power of thought and how it can work to our advantage. He wrote seven books on the subject at the turn of the twentieth century. The *Edinburgh Lectures on Mental Science,* perhaps his most popular edition, contains a brief discourse that sums up what he calls the "Train of Causation." To paraphrase: Everything begins with an *emotion or feeling,* which gives rise to a *thought;* the *judgment* then decides whether to materialize that thought. If the thought is approved by the judgment, the *imagination* is put into motion by visualizing that thought as already accomplished; the *will,* then, is exercised by holding that picture of the materialized thought until it manifests as a reality in your life.

This train of causation as described by Troward is important to psoriatics in that they can help the healing process by fixing their thoughts on the idea that their skin is already healed and visualizing it as an accomplished fact. Patients who follow through on all other measures, then add this power of visualization, have taken a giant step in ridding themselves of this disfiguring disease. The biggest obstacle to overcome is the patient's impatience. Unless he or she is willing to give the process time to work it will end in failure.

Troward emphasizes that once an idea is set in motion by our thoughts, its forward movement cannot and will not stop until the goal is achieved, unless we ourselves send out opposite, conflicting thoughts that neutralize or nullify our original thought.

Nothing could be clearer—or simpler. Nothing begins without a thought's setting it in motion. Hold on to the thought, and in ways beyond knowing, you will realize it at the appointed time. Do not become confused by trying to intellectualize how the process works. This is neither possible nor necessary. And the "train of causation" is available to all humanity. It is, in my opinion, the only explanation for the thought-provoking statement that "all men are created equal." This becomes more understandable to me when I add, "All men are created equal once they realize they have the power of thought at their command to set things in motion that work for them."

According to Troward, the very forces of the universe will gather to externalize the thoughts of a single human being. This is why warlords, feudal kings, early church officials, and self-proclaimed dictators kept the people subdued, either by force or by "divine" decree: they wanted to prevent the people from thinking! The United States of America became the greatest nation on earth in a mere two hundred years (as compared to other nations) because its people had freedom of thought.

You might be asking what all this has to do with psoriasis. It has a great deal to do with it when you realize that we are talking about a principle. The principle is "Thoughts are Things," and you have the power to set in motion the forces that bring all things into being, including the health of your body.

Let us put Troward's "train of causation" to practical use and apply the principle to the healing of psoriasis.

## The Thought Process

The process starts with a feeling or emotion to rid oneself of this disease. The *desire* is thereby established. Then, another part of our mental machinery comes into action, the *judgment,* meaning, you must determine whether you truly want to get rid of this psoriasis. (Some don't.) If, by your judgment, you decide, "I want the psoriasis cured," you have set the goal. Now, how can you attain that goal? By imagining it in your mind as already accomplished! This is done by using the *will* to direct the *imagination.* Simply stated, the will comes forward and directs the imagination to hold the picture of the desired end result. This plants a seed, so to speak, that, in time will continue to grow until the desired result is externalized. In this case, the goal is the appearance of clear, healthy skin.

The progressive building blocks needed to bring about the desired result may be: recognizing the necessary regimen, adhering to the diet, practicing internal cleansing, getting the spinal adjustments, faithfully taking the teas, and so forth.

It is most important to understand the relation of the will to the imagination. According to Troward, the function of the will "is to keep the imagination centered in the right direction. We are aiming at *consciously* controlling our mental powers instead of letting them hurry us hither and thither in a purposeless manner, and we must therefore understand the relation of these powers to one another for the production of external results."

Here is something worth memorizing and always keeping in mind: When the will and the imagination are in conflict with each other, the imagination always wins. In other words, if you cannot picture what you desire as accomplished, what you say or even shout over the rooftops is meaningless. I'll discuss this more later. At this point, it is necessary only to grasp the overall principle: what you visualize through the imagination will, in time, be realized.

## To Illustrate

One of the biggest hindrances I have encountered a few times in the healing process is the patient's inner belief (whether conscious or unconscious) that his skin disease must be a punishment from God. With such a belief harbored in the mind, it is nearly impossible to obtain positive results. As long as the patient believes he *deserves* to have psoriasis, he will succeed only in retaining the disease, for ridding himself of it would, according to his belief, be going against what he thinks is God's will. So even if help is readily available to him, he will avoid it to conform to his inner belief.

The story is told of a young prince of the Medici family in northern Italy, centuries ago, who was born with a crippled, deformed body.

Fortunately, he did not believe that the body he was born with was the "will of God," and at a very young age he determined to correct it by exercising the art of visualization. Because of his physical deformity, he avoided public communication and confined himself to an area within the palace grounds for his studies and meditations. Since he was a prince, he could have just about anything he wished. What the wise young man ordered would, even by today's standards, be considered eccentric at best and hardly recognized as anything other than wishful thinking.

In the middle of the court where he spent most of his waking hours, he ordered a statue to be carved by a leading sculptor of the day. The statue was to be a classic figure of a powerful Roman centurion—strong, stately, proud, and determined, but with one special feature: the head was to bear the likeness of the young prince. Month after month, year after year, the prince would continue to sit and meditate in his favorite gardens where the statue stood. He would see himself, as he wished he were, materialized in all his glory every day. With the passing of years, his subconscious mind gradually accepted the message, and the day came when the prince stood straight and strong, a magnificent specimen of manhood, an exact living replica of the model statue.

We learn from this story the power the mind holds over the body and that, in spite of all odds, the seemingly impossible can materialize. We also learn that the key is to picture in our mind's eye what we want. Whatever way we help ourselves to picture it is fine, as long as the desired result is achieved. We may, therefore, start our quest for beautiful clear skin with the happy certainty that God or the Creative Forces are on our side. First, we plant the seed, then water and take care of it, and then let it grow.

To those afflicted with psoriasis, Edgar Cayce offers help in visualizing the disease gone from their bodies by stating, "There is a cure." This completely refutes the age-old orthodox concept that there is no cure for psoriasis.

This is one important reason I often have my successful patients meet those just beginning the regimen. It is the most powerful incentive for them to take heart and realize that they can get well. It strengthens their will, which, in turn, directs the imagination to cling to that picture of perfect health. Then, by the law of attraction, their picture is materialized. One cannot set a time limit on how long it will take. Each person is a law unto himself. I can say with conviction that by following this method of "right thinking," you can realize your desire in the shortest, natural period of time. Staying on the "right" road of thinking requires a constant vigilance, a "guardian at the gate," if you will, to ward off the intrusion of destructive thoughts, statements, or gestures, which will distort, or even reverse, the thought patterns that spell success.

## Backfire!

An excellent example of practicing the "guardian at the gate" principle took place right in my reception room. Two new psoriasis patients met one evening at my office. Both were young women with severe cases of psoriasis. I introduced them to each other, as I have often arranged for patients to meet, in the hope that one would encourage the other. One patient, the positive one, was very enthusiastic at first and quickly began discussing the regimen with the other woman. It soon became apparent that the other woman did not share her enthusiasm, was filled with doubt, had a defeatist attitude about the entire matter, and thought nothing of transferring her discouragement to the patient who was trying to help her.

Later, when I met with the positive patient privately in the treatment room, I was immediately met with, "Dr. Pagano, I appreciate what you are trying to do, but please do not put me in the company of such a person again!" I was confused and rather embarrassed, to say the least, for having patients meet each other usually proves beneficial. Apparently, this situation was an exception. The positive patient voiced her dismay at the other woman's attitude and explained that she did not wish to be mentally "infected" by such thoughts. I explained that my purpose was for "*you* to encourage *her.*" She assured me she'd tried but soon realized that the other woman was not open to it. In fact, the opposite effect took place. Depression set in on the positive patient, while the other left the office clinging to her negativity.

About six weeks later the two women met again, purely accidentally, in my reception room. Their conversation seemed to begin where it had ended at their last meeting. The positive patient retained her composure while the other began her negative influence, even though her skin had shown improvement over the past month. This time, however, right in front of the other patients in the waiting room, the enthusiastic patient cupped her hands over her ears and said strongly and emphatically, "Please, I don't want to hear it!" Nevertheless, the other woman continued her negative remarks. Again, she was met with, "I just told you I do not want to hear any of your thoughts. Will you please stop!" Finally, when the message got across, the negative person saw she no longer had an audience and backed off.

In the treatment room, the positive patient said, "I'm sorry, Dr. Pagano, but that woman put me in such a depressed state for a month that I refuse to allow her to dump her garbage on me again!" I congratulated her on her forcefulness and determination to guard her mind from thoughts of a destructive nature. Hers was a perfect example of a person's choosing her thoughts rather than allowing thoughts from any source to enter her mind. Because she not only refused to allow such an attitude to be absorbed, but also counteracted it forcefully, her whole demeanor was changed. She was more cheerful, smiling, stronger, and determined to succeed. And succeed she did. Psoriasis is no longer a problem for her. She was so enthralled by the results that she wrote a lengthy letter to the head of dermatology at one of the country's leading psoriasis research centers, where she had previously been treated, relating her successful experience after years of suffering with the disease.

It must always be kept in mind that negative influences, of whatever nature, may appear very logical and realistic. At times, there are very strong arguments as to why something should *not* be followed. This is when patients need to be strongest in their resolve. People should keep before their mind's eye the successful cases, not the failures, and given time and patience, they will migrate toward a successful result. It may be likened to the man who did not know a thing couldn't be done, so he went ahead and did it. History abounds in true stories of successful outcomes of impossible feats. Add your name to the roster of successful outcomes in psoriasis cases and refuse to believe that "there is no cure." For many people, there most certainly is one!

Right thinking, therefore, is practiced successfully once you learn to recognize "wrong thinking" when it is directed at you. This may not be as easy as it sounds. There are many, often well-meaning, individuals who cast doubts on a patient's efforts. Their thoughts, usually in the form of remarks, can get a patient off track if that patient doesn't learn to recognize them. These subtle remarks include:

"I'll believe it when I see it."

"But there's no cure for psoriasis."

"Why waste your time?"

"Here, have another piece of cake"

Recognize these remarks for what they are—*destructive*! My patients know more about the course they are following than do the bystanders. It never fails to amaze me how some people presume to talk authoritatively without so much as reading a book on the subject or attending a lecture. If the patient, by necessity, is living with or is constantly in the presence of such people, then the best thing to do is follow an age-old philosophy: "Go and tell no man!" Get results first and tell them later. Success requires no explanation; failure permits no alibis.

## The Mental Formula of Émile Coué

At first glance, it would not surprise me to see a few raised eyebrows when I talk about a mental formula that can help anyone not only with his physical health, but with his outward circumstances as well. Does such a formula exist? The answer is an unequivocal yes. It was formulated by Émile Coué of France in the mid-nineteenth century. Devoting his life to the study of mental attitude in the healing or alleviation of disease, Coué gained considerable popularity because of his simple method of enlisting the aid of intangible healing forces.

Coué revealed a "secret" in which we can use the most powerful instrument in the world, our own mind, to help us. First, we must understand a bit about how our mind functions.

In brief, you must look upon your mind as two minds: the *conscious,* the faculty you are using at this very moment to read this book, and the *subconscious,* the faculty that is active when you are asleep or when the conscious faculty is subdued. There is a reciprocal action between the two minds; that is, the conscious mind can (and does) send suggestions to the subconscious mind and, if repeated often enough, the subconscious accepts it as true and brings it forth in your life. The subconscious does not have the power of reason. It accepts as true whatever is impressed upon it. The conscious mind, on the other hand, *does* have the power of reason. It can weigh things and decide what it will believe on the basis of the facts placed before it. The subconscious mind then receives the thought projection, once the conscious mind is convinced it is the way to go, accepts it as true, and eventually manifests it in your life.

Whether your personal circumstances are of a positive or negative nature, this is the process by which your subconscious mind works. Time and again, experiments in modern hypnosis have proven this to be the case. At present, hypnosis (or the better term *suggestive therapy*) has gained its rightful, respected place in modern medicine. The most valuable hypnosis, however, is the proper use of self-hypnosis. Through understanding and properly applying self-hypnosis to address your subconscious mind, you can make your life decidedly easier and more fruitful and healthful.

The key to effective self-hypnosis is *repetition.* By constantly repeating a phrase (mentally or verbally), the thought will eventually take hold and begin to manifest in your life. Some people write their desire on little cards and place them in strategic areas where they can view them occasionally. Another very helpful method is to make your own self-hypnosis tape recording and play it each night and every morning. An example of how some of my patients do it may be found in appendix C.

The first thing that must be dismissed from your mind is the notion that to practice self-hypnosis you must walk around like a half-dazed zombie. The exact opposite is true. You will be more alert and aware. The difference is that your mind will be subconsciously focused on a definite goal, and what the mind is centered on eventually becomes a reality. Again, it is not necessary for anyone to know the exact intricacies of how it works, any more than it is necessary to understand the workings of the internal combustion engine to drive a car. In both instances, we derive the benefits by learning how to turn the key and direct the power.

Turning the key toward good health is greatly enhanced when you understand that the thoughts you project into your subconscious mind eventually manifest in your physical body. Although this principle had existed since time immemorial, in modern times, it was Émile Coué who proved, beyond a doubt, that truly, you have direct power over the health (and disease) of your body. To some, this may seem to be a rash assumption. It is not. It is a fact of nature, your inherent birthright, your gift of the Divine!

Cognizant of this law, Émile Coué, after twenty years of experimenting, formulated a statement of a few words that, if practiced twenty times a day for twenty days, will enter one's subconscious realm and come forth in one's life. These most powerful words are: "Every day in every way, I am getting better and better." (*Note:* It does not indicate improvement in some dim, distant future. It states "I am," not "I am going to be." It makes clear the time is now, and although you may not be as healthy at the moment as you wish to be, you are becoming so.)

One stipulation, however, is brought out in Coué's works; that is, the affirmation must be within reason. Realistically, there may be a point of no return when, after abusing yourself with the wrong foods, attitudes, and emotions for so many years, the problem becomes irreversible. This is also stated in one of the Cayce readings. Even so, this should not deter or discourage a patient, for there are powers of mind that haven't even been tapped. New discoveries are made every day. What has never happened to anyone may happen to you.

To the beneficial formula, "Every day in every way, I am getting better and better," by Coué, I have added a few phrases that should help the psoriatic in particular:

"The diet is easy, nutritious, and cleansing."

"I have desire only for the foods that I know are healthful to me."

Write these sentences on an index card and keep it at your bedside. These words should be memorized and repeated as often as possible, especially just before you drift off to sleep and as soon as you begin to awaken in the morning, for these are the two periods of time when your subconscious mind is most amenable to suggestion. If, during the night, you find yourself semi-asleep and semi-awake, immediately repeat the suggestion. This period is known as the "muse" and will receive, and actually send, suggestions of guidance. Coué recommended that you whisper these suggestions so you can hear yourself say them. This is more powerful than just thinking them silently. He also suggested making a string of beads with twenty nodules on it to help you keep count, and repeating the statement twenty times before bedtime and twenty times as you awaken. This is but sending desirable thoughts into the realm of your subconscious. It is using the faculty of mind to aid you in the control, or even complete alleviation, of the disease. It is based on sound, proven psychological principles, and it is yours to use for your betterment.

I can already hear many of my readers say, "Doctor, I tried what you said. I repeated my desires twenty times a day for twenty days and things are not better. In fact, they are worse!" This is not an uncommon result. As Coué and Troward clearly stated, "When the *imagination* and the *will* are in conflict with each other, *the imagination always wins*!" In other words, just to repeat a phrase over and over again is worthless if you cannot see it, feel it, and be it in your imagination. To clearly *picture* it as already part of you is essential for its externalization.

Often, it has been said, and with sound reasoning, "Think only of what you want; not of what you don't want!" Why is this advised? I trust my readers now grasp the idea that we draw to ourselves the very thing our minds are centered on.

Thomas Troward in his classic work *The Hidden Power* describes this process as follows:

> But people say, "We have not found it so. We are surrounded by all sorts of circumstances that we do not desire." Yes, you *fear* them, and in so doing you *think* them; and in this way you are constantly exercising this Divine prerogative of creation by Thought, only through ignorance, you use it in a wrong direction. Therefore, the Book of Divine Instructions so constantly repeats "Fear not; doubt not," because we can divest our Thought of its inherent creative quality, and the only question is whether we shall use it ignorantly to our injury or understandingly to our benefit.

## Practicing the Art of Visualization: Alpha and Omega

We think in pictures, not in words. We use words to describe scenes, and from them we formulate a picture in our mind.

Being deeply involved in the field of fine art practically all my life, I have learned to visualize completed scenes long before I even place my initial sketch on the canvas. I know in advance where I am going and what I want to accomplish. When the final stroke of the brush is made on the canvas, it is the materialization of what I pictured in my mind and, much to my amazement, it is often better than I anticipated.

This principle of visualization carries over to every phase of our lives and to every accomplishment. It holds true, most decidedly, in the state of our physical bodies. A beautiful, well-toned body does not happen by chance. It must first be *desired,* then *visualized,* then *accomplished.* "Seeing" the desired result is the surest way of making it materialize. The means and methods to accomplish this will be given to you in stages as you advance in the regimen. This is where perseverance comes in. Philosophically, it is referred to as the "alpha and the omega"—the first and the last. It means the entire series of causation, from the first originating movement to the final and completed result.

The *alpha* is the thought and visualization that the skin can be healed; the *omega* is the materialization of the goal—the skin is healed. All steps necessary to accomplish that end (omega) will be revealed, and, if acted upon diligently, they cannot miss their mark, in time, in the vast majority of cases.

Visualizing your skin as pure and clear as you want it to be is not complicated. See it happen. The steps will then take place more easily, until one day your dream of clear skin will replace the reddened, scaly patches of psoriasis. I emphasize to the patient to feel encouraged when little areas of clearing begin to occur and to disregard the other massive lesions that have not, as yet, shown any change, for in time, they, too, will follow suit. Don't think of what's left; think of what left!

## Release from Bondage by Imaging

There is another dimension to the healing process: *imaging,* or the use of mental imagery. Far-reaching, indeed, are the implications of the active use of imaging in the regulation of your body, mind, and circumstances. Only recently has this concept been recognized and fostered by leading thinkers, although the principle has been in existence since time began.

Dr. Norman Vincent Peale, in his book *Positive Imaging,* informs us of the effectiveness of imaging:

> There is a powerful and mysterious force in human nature that is capable of bringing about dramatic improvement in our lives. It is a kind of mental engineering that works best when supported by strong faith. It's not difficult to practice; anyone can do it. Recently it has caught the attention of doctors, psychologists, and thinkers everywhere, and a new word has been coined to describe it. That word is IMAGING, derived from imagination. An image formed and held tenaciously in the conscious mind will pass presently, by a process of mental osmosis, into the unconscious mind. And when it is accepted firmly in the unconscious, the individual will strongly tend to have it, for then *it has you.* So powerful is the imaging effect on thought and performance, that a long-held visualization of an objective or goal can become determinative. Imaging is positive thinking carried one step further.

If we are what we are, and where we are, because of the things we imagine within ourselves, then we can be what we want to be, and where we want to be, by the very same law. The difference is that we are now aware of this fact of life and can use it on a conscious, intelligent level to make our lives what we will. Instead of just wishing, we imagine it so, and so it will become.

## Directing Your Thought

There are but two kinds of people in the world: those who say, "I can," and those who say, "I can't"—and they are both right. Does this sound contradictory? I assure you, it is not. You see, you draw into your life what you think about day in and day out. Think *health* and you draw it to you; think *illness* and that becomes your lot in life. In other words, you become what you think about, or as the author and mystic Manly Palmer Hall teaches, "The wise think health." It is more than a poignant saying; "it is an incontrovertible law."

The first thing that must be realized is that it *is* possible to be healed of psoriasis; it *can* be done. Then set in motion the law of expectancy—by visualizing healing as already accomplished. Little by little, day by day, as the law takes hold, improvement is noted, until the day comes when you are free of the malady. For the most part, psoriasis is indeed reversible, even in the most severe cases. It may require more discipline and time on the part of the patient and the doctor, but it can be done. That is what really matters. Although this principle has been with us since the dawn of history, it is now, at the brink of a new age, that we have become more cognizant of it. Since this concept is ours to use, why not use it? To put it succinctly, think only of what you want, not of what you don't want, for you will draw into your life what you think about. To think is to create; therefore, think health and you create it. This is what is meant by "right thinking."

## Let It Go!

In my opinion, there are a number of patients who, unknowingly, retain the disease even though they hate the thought of having it. I say "unknowingly" because this is carried out on the subconscious level. With some people, especially those who have had the disease for several years, completely ridding themselves of the disease may seem like taking away part of their personality, as they have long been identified with the disease, both in their own minds and in the minds of others. Don't fall victim to this trap! Get rid of it. Let it go. You don't need it!

There is only one way to change that destructive attitude: refuse to accept psoriasis as a part of your being. Remember always that we are a spirit with a body, not the other way around, and the spirit is pure by nature. So, from a psychological point of view, refuse to admit psoriasis into your private chamber (your mind and body). Cast it out! Evict it from your sacred home; it has no place there. If you must refer to it, say "psoriasis," not "my psoriasis." It is not yours, and what is not yours should not, cannot, really be a part of you.

## The Law of Expectancy

The final ingredient necessary to realize your desire is to set the wheels in motion with the underlying sense of *expecting* it to happen. If you don't do this, it will be as though you planned a dinner, invited your friends, prepared the food, bought the right wine, set the table, dressed to receive your guests, *and expected them to not show up*!

Does this make sense? Of course it doesn't. Having faith, as I see it, is having the awareness that your thought, by its very nature, has creative power. It is not something to be attained. It is! What is needed is not the power but the knowledge, the awareness that this is a built-in mechanism. It is used every day by everyone. How it is used can be determined by observing the end result.

# CHAPTER 11

# The Emotional Factor

Perhaps the question most commonly asked by psoriatics on their initial visit to the office is "Doctor, isn't psoriasis due to nerves?" And the answer is "Yes, it could be—but not always."

By "nerves" patients do not mean the anatomical nerve connections to and from the spinal column, as previously described. What they mean by nerves in this case is nervous tension, irritability, aggravation, stress, domestic or job pressure—in short, their feelings about things, their emotional state—the emotional factor.

Although you cannot see or measure emotions, you can certainly witness or experience their effects. In the case of psoriasis, it is negative emotions that could start the chain reaction, leading to hyperacidity in the system over an extended period of time, which can contribute to an eventual breakdown of the intestinal walls.

Throughout the Edgar Cayce works, we are constantly reminded to curb our hostilities toward others. You don't want to be a doormat, but holding grudges and ill feelings (even if apparently justified) only results in poisoning your own system. In fact, such attitudes can turn a body acidic even more readily than does eating the wrong foods.

Chemical analysis of the perspiration of criminals has proven that the secretions of the body undergo certain distinct changes under the influence of different emotions. It is possible to trace the existence of hidden anger, fear, grief, or remorse and distinguish one from the other, merely from this chemical difference in the fluids.

The perspiration of an angry man contains deadly poisons. More familiar is the fact that extreme fright or anger can poison or dry up the milk of a nursing mother, and even the lesser emotions of worry or annoyance will vitiate its quality. Violent grief or terror will so affect the pigment of the glands at the roots of the hair as to turn the hair white in a few hours. Good news brightens the eyes and straightens the stooping figure; bad news blanches the cheek and destroys the appetite. Confirmed invalids have many times found undreamed-of strength when obliged to meet some great emergency unaided.

Virgil said of his soldiers, "They are able because they *think* they are able," and Mulford's theory that the quality of thought determines the body's condition is well founded. This is no less true in nervous ailments than in others, but in these, it is more quickly and easily proven because of the close, direct relation between the brain and the nervous system.

The term *neurodermatitis* was coined in the year 1891 by two French physicians, Louis Brocq and Leonard Jacquet, to describe skin disorders that have their origins in emotional states. In the same year, a Russian scientist, A. G. Polotchoff, suggested that emotional upsets were sometimes among the causes of psoriasis.

Since then, research, especially by psychologically oriented dermatologists, has established that skin disorders often cause psychological problems and vice versa. One of my patients definitely traces the origin of his psoriasis to a painful divorce he experienced twenty years ago, even though he is happily married now. Another patient's psoriasis considerably improved after she married "Mr. Right." Yet another patient's psoriasis cleared when she divorced. What does all this tell us? It tells us, unmistakably, that our personal reaction to a situation determines the effect that particular situation has upon us.

Jane E. Brody, in her well-documented *New York Times* article of May 24, 1983, "Emotions Found to Influence Nearly Every Human Ailment," refers to the work of Dr. George F. Solomon, a University of California psychiatrist. "Mind and body are inseparable," he said. Brody wrote:

> The brain influences all sorts of physiological processes that were once thought not to be centrally regulated. The studies also show that the traditional concept of "stress" as a demanding life event,

is too imprecise to use as a measurement of how stress affects health. What is distressing to one person may be stimulating to another. Rather, the researchers are finding it is how a person responds to life events, not the events themselves, that influences susceptibility to disease. The studies indicate that failure to cope well with stress can impair a person's ability to fight off illness; whereas, adequate coping with a high-stress life may reflect "psychological hardiness" that is actually protective.

That we have within ourselves the power to *decide* our reaction to life's events is, to me, one of the most profound discoveries of our time, for it places our state of happiness (or misery) largely in our own hands. For instance, to be slighted, insulted or purposefully abused is to conjure up the most basic of human emotions—anger. Yet uncontrolled anger has caused pain and hardship to evolve by its accompanying state of hatred and resentment. The original cause, whether hurtful words or acts, is often lost, forgotten, or seen as inconsequential compared to the stormy aftermath.

Some readers may remember the gasoline shortage of 1973. Lines of cars at gasoline stations edged in front of one another, triggering violent tempers among drivers, physical harm, and even murder. Because of the hatred that ensued, mental poisons took over the minds of many motorists, which resulted in penalties in the form of legal fees, physical injuries, and even jail sentences.

Why did all this occur? Because of negative emotional states. Fortunately such extreme situations are rare. It is the everyday, relatively minor irritations that we must guard against. This does not mean we should become passive, impotent, slothful personalities. No one is asked or expected to remain in an abusive situation. Expressing yourself, even forcefully, is in keeping with sound mental health. The trick is not to carry inner resentments and condemnatory thoughts, for these can poison the blood, as mentioned previously. Make no mistake about it—the one who hates suffers internally more than the one hated. For one thing, the one who is hated is in many cases not even aware of it. But the one who hates is certainly aware of it day by day and experiences the aftereffects hate carries: an internal buildup of poisons, toxins, and acidity.

While I was an intern in Denver, Colorado, it was my pleasure and honor to personally meet one of the most renowned thinkers of our time, Manly Palmer Hall. His inspirational words from *Healing, the Divine Art* ring out on this subject as clearly today as they did then:

**The Negative Emotion of Fear—Fear Fixations and Phobias**
Another irrational emotion is hatred; defined as an intense form of dislike, it is far more dangerous to the one who hates than to the object of the hatred.

**No Health Where Hate Is—Hatred, the Irrational Emotion**
No one can hate and be healthy at the same time. It is essentially human for a person to dislike those who have injured him, filched his worldly goods, or frustrated his reasonable accomplishments. The other person's fault may be great, but the one who hates him, no matter how just the cause, has the fault which is the greater. The Scriptural admonition, to do good to those who despitefully use us, is not only a noble statement of spiritual truth, but a cardinal tenet of psychotherapy.

Conversely, the one who practices patience, gentleness, and kindness tends to experience the aftereffects of such attitudes: radiant health, cheerfulness, and joy. The triune principle of Mind, Body, and Spirit cannot be separated. Practice keeping the mind pure of prejudice, hatred, and jealousy, and the body responds with increased energy, vigor, and vitality. Keep the body cleansed internally and externally, flexible and active, and the mind reacts with enthusiasm, cheerfulness, and acuity.

To the person who justifies a negative attitude by saying, "But I can't help it, this is the way I am," I say, "Have you tried?" Did any of us know how to ride a bicycle when we were youngsters, before taking the necessary falls and lumps? Were we all born swimmers? No, we had to learn everything. That same principle applies to sports, or any other physical or mental activity as well as thinking processes. As far as your attitude is concerned, learn to think in a way that would best serve your interests. A different viewpoint may be all that's necessary. It has been demonstrated that a violent argument may be offset instantaneously by exercising a sense of humor. I can recall a true story of how a little old lady warded off a would-be mugger who confronted her on a dark street, gun in hand, with full intentions of robbing her of what little she had and possibly causing physical harm. When the thief jumped in front of her with his gun pointed at her face and demanded her purse, she responded with, "Oh, young man, what is the trouble? Can't you find a job? You know I don't blame you, finding a job is so hard these days. Is that a real gun? May I see it? I never saw a real one before." He answered, "Damn it lady, you got me all confused," and ran off into the night.

She did not respond in the way he anticipated. Panic, fear, and submission would have been the normal reaction. But confusion claimed the mind of the perpetrator because her reaction broke all the rules. By adopting a calm, serene attitude, the woman avoided being robbed and harmed, while at the same time prevented the mugger from committing a crime.

We must realize that to a very large extent, we have the power to control our reaction to whatever happens to us. To put it more succinctly, it is not what happens to us, it is what we think of what happens to us that determines our misery or happiness.

## Our Built-In Antennae

The idea that aggravating circumstances, or one's reaction to the circumstance, have a decided effect on the skin is nothing new to most psoriatics. One of my patients in particular has no problem relating to that concept. Afflicted for twenty years, he readily admits to experiencing all sorts of sensations on his skin, usually in reaction to job-related pressures. His skin practically screams at him when he is upset. Itching, tingling, blotching, and flare-ups are the immediate reactions. Although this patient follows all of the rules from a dietary point of view, his is a case where we both agree that his basic cause is emotional.

In an exceptionally informative article titled "Bringing Peace to Embattled Skin" (*Psychology Today*, February 1982), Ted A. Grossbart, PhD, a clinical psychologist at Beth Israel Hospital in Boston and in the Department of Psychiatry at Harvard Medical School, wrote, "The causes of skin disorders are varied. Heredity plays a role in some.

Bacteria, viruses, and physical and chemical irritants are important in others. Whatever the underlying cause, emotional problems may increase the frequency and severity of attacks. They may even be the fundamental cause of some disorders." Grossbart continued with, "The skin lives an emotional life of its own. It remembers, rages, cries, and punishes for real or imagined sins."

There is no question that we are dealing with a two-edged sword. The condition of the skin affects the emotions, and the emotions affect the skin. There is an interaction between the two that cannot be denied.

Fortunately, helping one often helps the other, which perhaps explains why we should try to keep our thoughts constructive. When the patient learns to control the emotions, the skin improves. When external applications help the skin, the emotions are decidedly affected, producing a more joyful, hopeful countenance. This is why I do not discourage sufferers, particularly those severely affected, from incorporating controlled ultraviolet light or other proven medical procedures to help clear the skin, if they so desire. It does not interfere with the regimen. If it helps a person feel better about himself, it is a plus. It is best, however, to continue with all the other measures as outlined. If and when UV light or some such therapy temporarily helps clear the skin, I emphasize that the patient should not be lulled into believing the problem is permanently resolved and that he or she can now safely discard the regimen.

## At Times a Paradox

There are people who, from all outward appearances, want to rid themselves of the disease, but when success is forthcoming, they retract and break the rules, thereby sabotaging their healing and *allowing* the disease to return. Undoubtedly they deny playing such a game. Nevertheless, in some cases, it is true. For years they may have been the center of attention, with sympathy and pity constantly showered upon them because of their dilemma. They *subconsciously* feel that ridding themselves of the disease is a threat to being the center of attention. They are in a mental quandary. On the one hand, they want to be cured; on the other, they fear they will lose that prize we all desire—attention. When they come to grips with this paradox and see it for what it is, they usually improve.

Moreover, having the disease has become such a habit that some people cannot visualize themselves without it. But they must, or the results will be slight or nonexistent. They must get rid of the "old friend" as they would an "old sore."

There are those who also feel they must retain the disease as a form of self-punishment for reasons only they know. Whether they deserve such punishment is beside the point. The fact is they *think* they do, so they become their own judge and jury. I try to tell such people to be kinder to themselves and to take life easier.

## A Positive Twist

Stressful situations are usually linked to negative circumstances. We often connect ulcers, headaches, nervousness, and conditions such as indigestion to an unhappy situation. Perhaps it is our working conditions, a love affair that has gone sour, family strife, or school pressures. We must also recognize the fact that stressful feelings can come from joyful occasions that may also have a deleterious effect upon the person involved, depending on his or her attitude. For instance, one patient was doing extremely well with her psoriatic arthritic condition when suddenly there was a flare-up of the arthritis in her joints, although her skin remained clear. We went over all aspects of the regimen to see if she was inadvertently violating parts of the principles of treatment. She was not. It came out later in the conversation that she had just become engaged to be married, a few days before the flare-up occurred. When I asked if she thought this placed her under an emotional strain even though it was a joyous occasion, she quickly nodded yes. This was the only explanation we could come up with, and she fully appreciated its implication.

At first glance this story may seem to be a contradiction in terms, but I assure you it is not. You see, it was not the joyous occasion that triggered this woman's arthritis but the *worry* that accompanied the event, even though happiness underlined the whole situation. Again, let us be mindful that it is not the emotional experience that determines our physical reaction; it is our *attitude* toward the occurrence that directs our response.

## The Mind Worketh Miracles—or Misery!

I often recall a conversation I had with a patient while at the hospital in Denver. It closely parallels this type of reaction but to a much more devastating degree. This gentleman had been working at a well-known department store for several years. His goal was to become a department manager, and for years he strove for it in every possible way. Then the day arrived. He was notified that as of a certain date, he would take over the entire department as manager. The next morning, the man could not get out of bed. A form of hysterical paralysis crippled his entire body. It was subsequently diagnosed as spastic multiple sclerosis. It was a progressive disease with no hope for a cure.

Here is a situation where a man was advanced to the position he strove for and apparently desired, but in his case, much to his dismay and for reasons that may never be known, his physical reaction resulted in a severe illness. Was it because of a subconscious fear of what the new job entailed? For someone else, the reaction would be different, but to him, it was obviously more than he could bear. Perhaps it was the final straw that triggered an underlying disease process already in the making.

## On the Brighter Side

For approximately two years, it was my good fortune to have as my evening secretary a most delightful young woman whom I will call Judy. A most attractive, friendly, and energetic girl of eighteen, Judy held three jobs at one time, attended school, and was quite popular in her circle of friends. She had a problem, though—psoriasis.

After graduation, Judy decided to go out west to work on a ranch as a waitress. She sent out several résumés and finally decided on a beautiful dude ranch in northern Colorado. It would be her first time away from her home on the East Coast. Needless to say, Judy had the normal feeling of anxiety, knowing she would be on her own for the first time, in a strange place surrounded by new faces, thousands of miles from home.

Judy left for Colorado in her little car, with her luggage, her cowboy hat, and her psoriasis.

In early September I planned a vacation in Wyoming with the thought that I might be able to stop at the ranch where Judy worked and surprise her. Well, I did surprise her, but not half as much as she surprised me.

After our emotional greeting at the ranch and hours of stories of her great experiences, expressing her enthusiasm for her work and the land, she spoke of her *former* problem of psoriasis. I was amazed to see that there wasn't a mark on her. She related that she did take the saffron tea and slippery elm fairly regularly but was not, and could not be, totally strict with the diet.

When I asked about the reason for such a dramatic result, she answered without the slightest doubt, "It's my contentment." She was so inwardly happy with the conditions and her environment that she no longer produced her own poisons due to stressful feelings. Was it living with her parents that caused this strained feeling? Hardly. Judy was trying to get them to move out west as well, which they seriously contemplated.

Obviously, I do not recommend that anyone pick up stakes and change residence to rid himself of psoriasis. This, however, is what happened in Judy's case. Each person's psoriasis may have an entirely different cause. The goal is to seek out the cause of the particular condition and do everything possible to change it.

## A Triune Comparison

When we take the time to examine the teachings of three giants in their respective fields and find that they come to the same conclusion on the effect joy or anger has on the human organism, I, for one, want to pay attention, listen, and learn.

Compare the following:

**Francis M. Pottenger (scientific):** "Such emotions as fear, anger, and pain, act upon the sympathetics as shown by Cannon and his coworkers, while joy and happiness tend to preserve the normal physiologic nervous and endocrine equilibrium."

**Manly P. Hall (philosophic):** "Harmony in the mind results in the increasing health of the body; and harmony in the body improves the disposition of the mind."

**Edgar Cayce (spiritual):** "Anger causes poisons to be secreted by the glands [adrenals principally]. Joy has the opposite effect." (All the glands are involved to some extent.)

Could it be any more clear? These examples should answer the question of whether man should engage in "the pursuit of happiness." My belief is he should indeed, for then and only then is he living in his natural state. It should come as no surprise to him, however, if he finds that his pursuit originates and terminates within his own self.

## What You "See" Is What You Get

Can the mind have such an effect as to create a skin reaction by either actual or imaginary irritants? It most certainly can. An eye-opening incident took place when two Japanese physicians, Y. Ikemi and S. A. Nakagawa, experimented with a plant similar to poison ivy. After placing a patient under hypnosis, they applied the poison leaf to the skin with the added suggestion that it was harmless. There was no skin reaction. Conversely, if a leaf that was harmless was placed on the skin with the suggestion that it was toxic, a decided reaction took place. The patient's skin became red and irritated. The subconscious mind of the patient did not argue the point. It accepted the suggestion as truth and reacted accordingly. (This theme is covered in the previous chapter). For now, suffice it to say that the mind, through thought or emotion, can and does affect skin reactions.

## A Possible Solution

The causes of our emotional makeup are not always obvious. They could be so deep-rooted within our subconscious that only long, arduous self-analysis or professional help may provide some answers.

My personal conclusion, based on a lifetime of observing "successful" personalities versus "losers," is that the answer lies largely in the vision we have of *ourselves*. Do you like what you see in the mirror? If you don't, you have another job to do other than clear your skin.

You must start today to appreciate yourself in a healthy, divinely inspired way, not as one on an ego trip. This means to like the kind of person you are and be at peace with your inner self.

What if you don't like the kind of person you are? Then start doing something that will help you like the person you are. Do something for somebody else. Through the ages, the most frequent advice regarding physical and mental health is to adopt the attitude of helping others. This is not all that difficult. It does not require earth-shattering demonstrations. All it takes is being kind and gentle, just being patient, *first* with yourself and then with others.

It is the little everyday things, common to all of us, that make for the realization of this principle. We can't all be an Albert Schweitzer serving the sick and depressed in the wilds of Africa or a Mother Teresa administering to the needy in the slums of Calcutta. For one thing, theirs were inspirationally guided missions that came from the very depths of their souls. Unless this same inner guidance does the directing, the end result would be pure mimicry and probably end in dismal failure. It is in the world around us—our families, neighbors, friends, associates—where those little kindnesses find their meaning and expression.

## Activate Your Higher Power

You cannot separate emotions from religious beliefs. The question before us is whether religious beliefs can play a part in healing disease. A study of four thousand elderly people living at home, conducted in 1996 by the National Institute on Aging, found that "those who attend religious services are less depressed and physically healthier than those who don't attend or who worship at home."

In other words, belief in a higher power stimulates that "higher power" to act in your behalf. Ignore it, and it will ignore you in turn, for nothing is forced upon you. It is there, waiting only for your recognition and direction. It is there for you to use or abuse. You don't have to be a rocket scientist to put it in motion. All it takes is your awareness of its existence; then it's up to you to derive its benefits, whether on a general level or a cellular level. It permeates every atom in space; it is the force that runs in, around, and through us.

Edgar Cayce, in the book *Search for God,* states, "Influences from within are stronger than from without; thus, our higher selves stand ready to help, if we are really anxious to set ourselves right."

## Helping Yourself and Others at the Same Time

Is there something we can do on a daily basis that can in some way be a blessing to ourselves and to those around us? Yes, there is—something that is so simple that it often evades us: smile!

There's an old philosophy that has weathered the test of time: "To become, act as if." It means, if you want to be happy, act as if you are happy, and in ways beyond knowing, the *spirit* of happiness will find its way into your soul and heart. Like anything else, it takes practice, but in time, the technique will pay off, and you will find it works in many areas of life, if given a chance. One of the best methods of feeling a glow of happiness within is to smile, "even if it takes the hide off," as Cayce says.

Have you ever noticed how people in general tend to gravitate to the person who smiles? I believe the reason for this is that people who smile project an image of a person who has risen emotionally above it all. Did you ever see a president of the United States who didn't smile—especially in recent years? A smile indicates an inner strength, that a person's feathers are not easily ruffled, that they have a sense of humor toward life. Other people subconsciously want that attitude to rub off on them.

I had this experience when I personally had the honor of meeting the Dalai Lama after my talk on psoriasis in Bangalore, India. His pleasing countenance was contagious; he was always smiling! He came to the United States in 1990 after receiving the Nobel Peace Prize and, in an interview, emphasized the importance of smiling.

# CHAPTER 12

# The Crowning Glory

Psoriasis on the scalp is one of the most unsanitary, uncomfortable, and unpleasant manifestations of the disease, and the self-consciousness a person develops because of its visibility makes it all the more disturbing. Through the years, I have worked out a hair treatment and a shampoo that have proven to be quite effective in ridding the scalp of accumulating scales, as well as enhancing the healing of the surface cells. Keeping in mind that the real healing comes from within, my patients' comfort and external appearance have been improved by following the treatment outlined at the end of this chapter. In severe cases, where there is a thickening of the scalp and heavy scaling, an electric heat cap treatment is employed. In less serious cases, a regular shampoo treatment is helpful, and the electric heat cap treatment is made optional.

At first glance, the routine may look bothersome, but I urge my patients to try these treatments at least once or twice. They soon realize that the procedures are quite simple, and once they understand them, they breeze right through them. To those who insist on using hair dyes and artificial coloring, I can only say, make a choice. You cannot get rid of the psoriasis and the gray hair simultaneously—at least not until the condition clears up.

## Does Psoriasis Cause Hair Loss?

There is no question that psoriasis on the scalp can and does cause hair loss, particularly if the lesions become too thick. For some people, hair loss becomes a major concern when they find their hair falling out in clumps. When you realize that the hair follicles extend only a fraction of an inch into the subcutaneous cellular tissue of the scalp, it is easy to understand that hair loss is not only possible but can be expected when psoriasis affects the deeper layers of the skin. This is why the scalp should be shampooed *gently* with the fleshy part of the fingertips rather than the nails. There is one encouraging note: in the majority of cases that I have treated, the hair grew back completely as the internal cleansing process took place.

One of my patients, a college student with a devastating case of generalized psoriasis and considerable hair loss, surprised me with a quick visit during his summer vacation to show me how well he was doing. Except for a few minor spots near the lower rib cage and a small area on his back, he was virtually clear of the lesions, which, at one time, had covered most of his body. For a few months he had neglected drinking his saffron tea, but he knew that once he resumed drinking it on a regular basis, the problem would rectify itself. I noted that he had trimmed down considerably, looked healthy and strong, and had a crop of thick hair.

He explained that the regrowth of his hair was one of his greatest joys, for when the disease was at its peak, he had been losing his hair by the handful. The only areas that did not regenerate were those he picked at, thus destroying the root of the hair follicle. This is certainly understandable, for if the root is preserved, the shaft of the hair can regenerate completely.

This patient, along with many others I have treated through the years, is a living example of how hair can grow back. Therefore, I advise my patients not to despair if psoriasis on the scalp is causing hair loss. It is possible that the hair can come back, in all its glory, healthier and stronger than ever.

## Psoriasis along the Hairline

Three products stand out above all others as having a beneficial effect for psoriasis along the hairline, the back of the ears, and in small, circumscribed areas on the scalp. They are Baker's P&S Liquid, medicated Vaseline, and Ray's Ointment. Although covered previously in chapter 9, I feel these products deserve to be mentioned again. They may be applied with the fingertips, cotton swabs, or a cotton-wrapped orangewood stick. They are to be rubbed in deeply but gently, taking care not to cause damage with fingernails. Remember, the skin is traumatized enough already.

## For Itchy Scalp

It may be hard to believe, but these common household mouthwashes are among the best products available to relieve itching of the scalp: Lavoris, Listerine, and Glyco-Thymoline. By rubbing them gently into the scalp in cases of dandruff or scaling, considerable relief can be immediate. These mouthwashes can also soothe a scalp that has flared up after an electric heat cap and oil treatment.

In the case of generalized itch all over the scalp, the mouthwashes may be diluted in a quart of warm water and used as a rinse, or they may be applied full strength, with the fleshy part of the fingertips, to specific itchy spots. Another anti-itch remedy used successfully by several of my patients is a mixture of two ounces of apple cider vinegar or white vinegar to six ounces of lukewarm water. It is mixed, slowly poured over the entire head, rubbed in gently and then left on for about a minute or two. It is rinsed with lukewarm water, followed by a final rinse of water as cool as is comfortable.

*Above all, do not scratch.* This can lead only to spreading of the psoriatic lesions, bleeding, and possibly infection.

## Shampoo and Electric Heat Cap Treatments

The shampoo treatment and an electric heat cap treatment that I have worked out for my patients are detailed in the following sections.

### Shampoo Treatment for a Scaly Psoriatic Scalp

My patients are directed to perform this once or twice a week or as deemed necessary.

### Necessary Items

- A large cake of Cuticura soap or a bottle of Cuticura shampoo (pre-ferred), tea tree oil shampoo, an olive oil–based shampoo, T-Gel, or Z-Tar shampoo
- An unlined shower cap (or a disposable one)
- One Handi Wipe or absorbent cotton strips
- An 8-ounce measuring cup
- A timer
- One bottle of apple cider vinegar (for thick hair) or white vinegar (for fine hair) or fresh lemons (alternative)

Psoriatic patients should never use any form of color or dye on their hair, especially when sores and scales are prevalent on the scalp, as this may very well cause an inflammatory, allergic, or even infectious reaction. Therefore, the following instructions for shampoo treatment should be applied only to the natural scalp.

Because of adverse effects on several patients who used a blow dryer or other hair dryer, I advise my patients not to use such electrical appliances. If they must be used, however, they should be used on the lowest or coolest setting. It is preferable that the hair be allowed to dry naturally.

### Shampoo Treatment

1. Wet hair thoroughly with warm water.
2. Massage the scalp, working the shampoo into a rich lather using the fingertips, not the fingernails.
3. Leave the lather on the scalp for a full three minutes, then rinse.
4. Repeat steps 1 through 3, then dry the hair with a thick towel.
5. For a final rinse, mix 2 ounces of apple cider vinegar, white vinegar, Lavoris, or Listerine with 6 ounces of lukewarm water, then gently work through the scalp.
6. Towel-dry the hair, and if you must use a hair dryer, use the "cool" setting.

This treatment may be repeated two or three times per week, depending on the thickness of the scales that accumulate on the scalp. Shampooing every day is not a good idea.

### Electric Heat Cap and Oil Treatment

Perform this treatment about twice a month, or as deemed necessary.

### Required Items

- An electric heat cap (available at health and beauty aid stores)
- Olive oil–peanut oil mixture (50/50), unscented
- Baby shampoo
- Apple cider vinegar, white vinegar, Lavoris, or Listerine
- An 8-ounce measuring cup

### Procedure for Treatment

1. Shampoo the scalp as described in steps 1 through 3 of the shampoo treatment.
2. After rinsing, towel-dry the hair without rubbing the scalp.
3. Cover the scalp with the olive oil–peanut oil mixture, gently massaging into the scalp (using the fingertips, not the fingernails) for about three minutes.
4. Place the heat cap over the scalp, using medium heat for twenty minutes, or less for very sensitive scalps.
5. Remove cap. You may leave on the coating of oil for a while, making sure to wipe off any excess with a good quality paper towel.
6. Wash the oils out with baby shampoo. To completely remove the oils, a second shampoo may be necessary.
7. For a final rinse, mix 2 ounces of apple cider vinegar, white vinegar, Lavoris, or Listerine with 6 ounces of lukewarm water, then gently work through the scalp.

Mouthwashes such as Lavoris, Glyco-Thymoline, and even Listerine, when rubbed gently into the scalp, can be beneficial in treating cases of dandruff or scaling or the flare-ups that may occur after an oil treatment. They have also been suggested for use in combating severe itching of the scalp.

## The Overnight Oil Treatment

Psoriasis of the scalp responds very well to the olive oil–peanut oil overnight application. After shampooing the scalp, as previously described, the patient then gently massages a 50/50 mixture of olive oil and peanut oil (such as Aura Glow or Almond Glow, or make your own), thoroughly into the scalp. A disposable shower cap is worn overnight. If it is more practical to do so, it can be left on for a few hours only before bedtime. In the morning, the cap is removed and the scalp shampooed to clean off the oil. Just a quick cleansing will do, followed by a rinse using two ounces of apple cider vinegar, Listerine, or Glyco-Thymoline in six ounces of warm water, or to make it more dilute, mix four ounces in twenty-eight ounces of warm water, making a full quart. Pour it over the scalp slowly and let it set for a minute or two, then make a final rinse using lukewarm or even cool water. The patient then pats the hair dry with a towel. You may use a blow dryer, but remember to use the "cool" setting.

Many effective shampoos exist today that were not available at the time of the first printing of this book. It is obvious that some work better on different people, so a person must try different shampoos to find out which is best for him or her. The following are products most frequently suggested to my patients:

- Olive oil shampoo (from Baar Products and the Heritage Store, see appendix D)
- Tea tree oil shampoo (from Baar Products and the Heritage Store)
- Neutrogena (T-Gel and T-Sal)
- Tegrin shampoo
- P&S shampoo (Baker's)
- Aloe vera gel shampoo
- Cuticura soap or shampoo (from Baar Products)

Baar Products has available a Psoriasis Kit that contains Slippery Elm Bark, American Yellow Saffron Tea, Psoriasis Medicated Scalp and Body Wash, and Psoriasis Cream. See appendix D for contact information.

The best results are obtained by leaving the soapy lather on the scalp for a few minutes before washing out. A second lather is applied and again allowed to stand for a few minutes before rinsing. Towel dry hair and do not use a hair dryer unless it is on the cool setting.

Some people report good results in removing scales on the body by using the lathered shampoo on all body lesions after the scalp has been lathered up. They then leave it on for a few minutes before washing off.

Oftentimes, I have seen a terribly afflicted scalp clear up before any other part of the body, with all hair restored to normal. In one particular case, a patient had a scalp with lesions that felt like golf balls. The lesions completely disappeared in about two months, once he committed himself to the regimen, after having suffered for years with the affliction.

Remember, try not to scratch the scalp. It can only lead to damage to the hair follicles and production of new lesions.

Carbolated Vaseline, which I recommended in this book's previous edition be applied to the hairline, can no longer be obtained. It had been used effectively for decades. It reminds me of a comment made by the great comedian George Burns in the movie *Going in Style*. He asked a pharmacist for a certain prescription he had been renewing for years and was told it was no longer available. Burns replied, "That figures—it worked!" In place of Carbolated Vaseline for the hairline, I suggest medicated Vaseline, available through your local pharmacy, or Ray's Ointment, available through the Heritage Store.

These topical remedies all help the scalp to feel better, but remember, the real healing comes from within.

## Psoriasis of the Face

It goes without saying that a person with psoriasis of the face agonizes over two things: (1) he has psoriasis, and (2) it is highly visible. This, along with psoriasis of the nails, will send the sufferer on an urgent quest to get it corrected, if possible, at any cost. If the alternative route outlined in this book is taken long enough, chances are good that the psoriasis will clear up anywhere and everywhere. That includes the face and the nails. The following, however, should interest you.

One day I received a phone call from a patient of mine whom I had not seen for about ten years. She related that she had done fine on the regimen, but for the past several months the psoriasis had broken out on her face. She was mortified. The outbreak was accompanied by a seemingly unrelated problem: a pungent, foul underarm odor. It was so bad that her fellow workers could not stand to be near her. She started using a powerful underarm antiperspirant instead of a deodorant. She used it extensively and persistently and managed to cover up the foul odor that emitted from under her arms. Then, suddenly, psoriasis broke out on her face. This woman, not thinking there was a connection, continued to use the antiperspirant. The condition on her face worsened.

Then she went on vacation to the tropics. Upon arriving and unpacking, she realized she had forgotten her antiperspirant. She panicked. What could she do since there was none to be found on the remote island? She simply had to resort to plain soap and water and the clean salt water of the Caribbean. To her amazement, the psoriasis on her face completely disappeared within seven days. Although the sun and salt water may have helped, she did not attribute her success to that. She offered her own explanation. She believed that the antiperspirant (which has aluminum in it) sealed off the pores of the skin under her arms, which prevented the normal toxins from exiting through that area. "The toxins had to go somewhere," she said, "so they chose to make their way up through the face." Once she removed the blockages that sealed off the pores, the toxins had a chance to exit the body as they were supposed to. She is satisfied with this explanation, and so am I.

I now suggest to all my psoriasis and eczema patients to use plain soap and water or a good deodorant without any antiperspirant. This may also have an effect on psoriasis of the scalp.

# CHAPTER 13

# Psoriasis on the Hands, the Feet, and the Nails

After giving it considerable thought, I concluded that psoriasis on the hands, the feet, and the nails deserved a chapter devoted solely to those portions of the body for two reasons:

1. Psoriasis on the hands, the feet, and the nails has long been recognized as one of the most treatment-resistant forms of the disease.

2. More demands are placed on the hands, the feet, and the nails than on any other part of the human anatomy. To be afflicted with psoriasis on these areas can be more devastating than having it anywhere else on the body, except for the relatively rare instance when it appears on the face. This is true from a visual as well as a mechanical point of view with regard to the hands. The effects of weight bearing make lesions on the feet excruciatingly painful.

People with psoriasis on the hands are extremely self-conscious and do whatever they can to avoid exposing their hands during business or social engagements. True, psoriasis is not contagious, but how many people know that? Or even care? They look upon it as unsightly and possibly contagious, so the sufferer feels compelled to hide his hands as much as possible. In the case of psoriasis on the feet, even though the feet are not ordinarily exposed, the awkward, pained gait one assumes is a dead giveaway that all is not right.

The following measures have proven with my patients to be very effective for psoriasis of the hands and the feet:

1. Soak the hands or the feet in a comfortably hot Epsom salts bath, preferably in a home whirlpool, for twenty minutes.

2. Pat dry and immediately massage warm peanut oil (or a combination of peanut oil and olive oil) well into the hands or the lower limbs and the feet, whatever the case may be. Castor oil can be used in the same way with equal effectiveness, as can Vaseline cocoa butter or coconut oil.

3. Place a small plastic bag over the hands or the feet after they have been massaged, and put on white gym socks. Or eliminate the bags and use only the gym socks. Leave the socks on for at least thirty minutes or, better yet, overnight.

## On Very Difficult Cases

When the scales are very hard, sharp, and crusty on the soles and the heels of the feet, I have advised the following, with very gratifying results. (This procedure may also be used on the palms of the hands, which, at times, can become as coarse as canvas.)

### Necessary Items
- Epsom salts
- Peanut oil
- Sodium bicarbonate (baking soda)
- Castor oil
- Small plastic bags or cotton or disposable plastic gloves
- White gym socks

### Procedure
1. Begin by bathing the hands or the feet in a comfortably hot Epsom salts bath, preferably in a whirlpool for fifteen to twenty minutes.

2. Massage warm peanut oil into the affected areas.

3. After the oil is absorbed, make a paste of sodium bicarbonate (baking soda) and castor oil and massage it into the affected areas.

4. Place plastic bags over the feet, followed by white gym socks, and leave these on for at least one-half hour, or better yet, over-night. The same procedure applies to severely affected hands. For the hands, disposable plastic gloves may be used, if desired. Remember, the plastic bags may be eliminated in favor of using only the white gym socks for both the hands and the feet, after they have been massaged with the oils. As discussed in chapter 9, the plastic wrap or plastic gloves may cause an irrita-tion under the skin in both psoriasis and eczema cases because of the sweating it causes.

If the Epsom salts bath and/or the baking soda and castor oil mix-ture prove to be too irritating to open sores, wash the hands or the feet off in plain warm water and avoid using this procedure until the cracks and sores heal over. In such cases, my advice is to use only plain warm water in the whirlpool, followed by a massage with peanut oil or castor oil only (without the baking soda), and then to cover with a bag and/or a sock. This is to be followed until the underlying sores and cracks are healed over.

In the spring of 2007, a young girl came into my office with severe psoriasis of the feet. Her feet were literally raw! She followed through on all of the above measures, and results were steady but extremely slow. Then, her feet suddenly cleared when she least expected them to. Why? She stopped eating bagels! She did not realize how constipating they were to her. When she stopped eating them, all of the prescribed measures kicked in and did their job unencumbered by backups in the bowel. The high gluten content in bagels renders them constipating. The moral of the story is, stay away from bagels!

## When Washing Dishes

It is best to use rubber gloves when washing dishes. Contact with dishwashing or laundry detergent can cause fiery irritation in psoriatic or eczematous skin. Sometimes, however, the rubber gloves themselves can cause such irritation, even if they are on for only a few minutes. If this occurs, cotton gloves should be worn under the rubber gloves.

## Two Success Stories

Two of the most severe cases of psoriasis on the hands and the feet that I have ever encountered are those of S.R., and B.K. (see the photos in this chapter).

S.R. was a fine young man who had suffered with this problem for seventeen of his nineteen years. Throughout his life, no expense was spared by his devoted parents in their search for effective remedies. None was found. All of his much-loved sports activities were curtailed or became impossible to perform. His social life was always under a cloud. He would avoid shaking hands with male friends and rarely attempted to hold a girl's hand. It took from four to six months, but S.R.'s hands and feet became as smooth as silk, with not a lesion or an abrasion to be found on them. He followed instructions precisely, and he was able to tell his encouraging story at a lecture I delivered at Virginia Beach.

S.R. made it very clear that diet appeared to be the culprit in his particular case. Tomatoes, he discovered, played havoc with his hands and feet. Since he had psoriasis only on those areas of the body, he made a concerted effort to get relief from the external effects of the condition. Adhering strictly to the recommendations, he would first soak his feet (or hands) in an Oster whirlpool massager. I recommend this unit above all others, as it has several cycles and keeps the water quite warm. It is a most valuable investment for a patient with this problem. After about fifteen or twenty minutes of soaking in the hot whirlpool, S.R. would pat his feet dry, and while they were still warm and even red from the treatment, he would saturate all the affected areas with the olive oil–peanut oil mixture or castor oil and massage it deeply into the skin. After a few minutes of massaging, being very generous with the oils, he would place a large plastic bag over each foot, followed by a clean white gym sock, and retire for the night. In the morning, he would remove the socks and the bags, wash his feet thoroughly, and then dress for the day and go about his business. Sometimes he would apply a light coating of castor oil to his feet, cover them again with plastic bags and gym socks, and leave these on, even at work.

His remarkable recovery, with complete regeneration of the surface epithelium of both feet, is vividly shown in the photographs below and on page 185. His hands cleared up simultaneously by means of the same procedure. His story, among others, is an inspiration to all psoriatics.

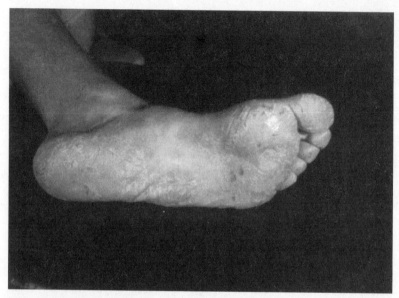

S.R., age 22, afflicted 18 years, at the start of the regimen.

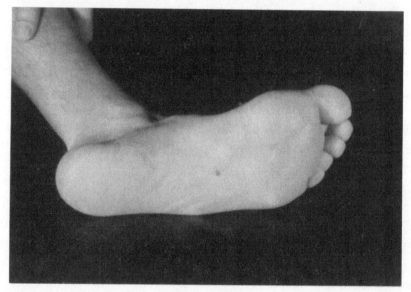

S.R., 10 months later.

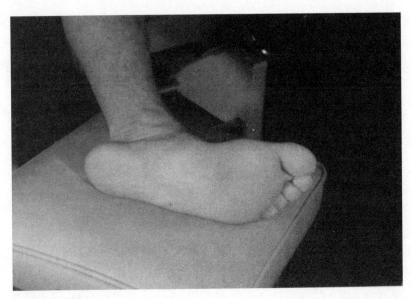

S.R., 5 years later.

Another case of remarkably quick and complete healing was that of B.K. (see the illustrations on page 186). Her psoriasis was all over the body, but most severe on the soles and heels of her feet, to the point that she could not even have bedsheets touch her skin. It was so painful that she had to have friends support her under the arms for her to walk into my office. As previously described, cases as severe as this call for covering the feet with a poultice of castor oil and baking soda after the initial soaking. This method of treatment was continued until all areas softened, and then only pure castor oil or the olive oil–peanut oil mixture was used. Bags and socks were placed over the feet every night, and areas that had been covered with razor-sharp scales became smooth and clear in a few months.

Several years later, I followed up to see how B.K. was doing. Her answer was "No problem!" If and when she has a flare-up, she places herself back on the regimen, and the slight recurrence disappears. In other words, her life is in order and has been ever since her initial clearing. In her case, the dietary culprits proved to be tomatoes, shellfish, and vinegar. Eleven years later, this patient remains in control of the disease.

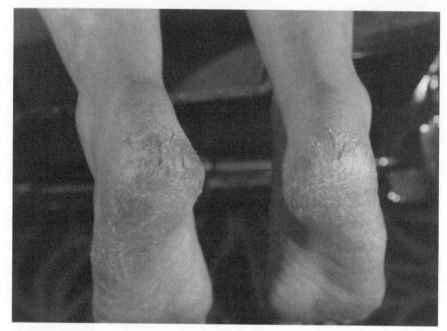

B.K, age 50, afflicted 2 years, at the start of the regimen.

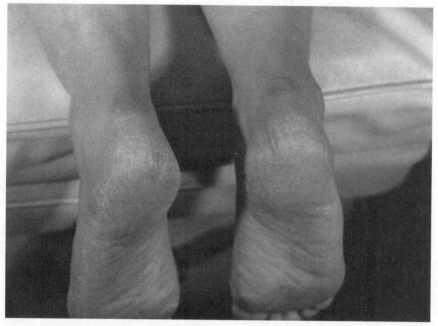

B.K., 5 months later.

## An Inspiring Case

It is well established that psoriasis of the hands and the feet is the most difficult type to clear up, since we are always on our feet and constantly using and abusing our hands. I find it most amazing to see people with this condition *only* on the palms of the hands and the soles of the feet. The reason for this is anybody's guess, but for one reason or another, this is the path the body has chosen to discharge its toxins.

In the past few years, we have found two additional external measures to help heal over the psoriatic lesions on the hands and the feet. Aquaphore has been on the market for several years and is available in most drugstores and can be ordered. It is used in the same manner as the other external applications, including the hydrophilic ointment with castor oil or the olive oil–peanut oil mixture, baking soda combined with castor oil if lesions are very thick, Vaseline, and so forth. Simply massage it in well after the hot soaks or whirlpool baths, cover with plastic wrap, put on a white sock, and leave it on overnight or at least several hours.

The other effective product is Bag Balm, an old farmer's product for keeping a cow's udder soft and pliable as well as preventing infection. It is applied similarly to the other external applications.

For a perfect example of how effective these procedures are, look at the pictures of K.B. on pages 188–189 and observe the results obtained in her severe case of pustular psoriasis-eczema on the hands and feet.

Recovery did not happen overnight, but in K.B.'s own words, "The diet was still the key factor in healing, combined with the external applications. It was well worth the effort." As an added bonus, she lost a total of forty pounds, a very welcomed side effect.

## A Word of Caution

Once clearing of the hands, especially the palms, has taken place, the patient must not make the mistake of abusing them through rough manual activity. Remember, the surface cells are new. The deeper layer, the dermis, is just beginning to come back to life. These areas need time to fully recuperate from the ordeal they have been through, perhaps for many years.

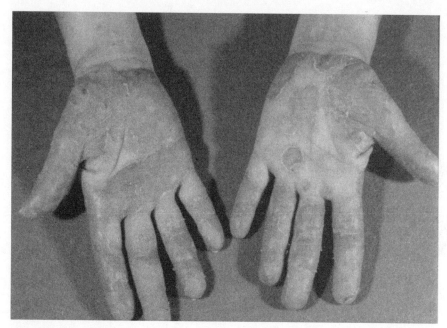

K.B., at the start of the regimen.

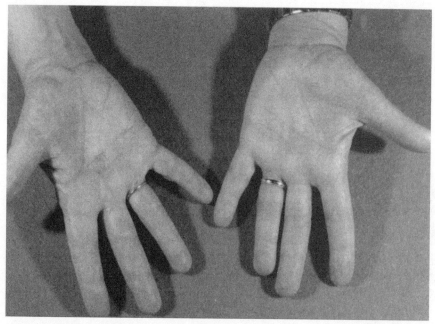

Patient K.B., 10 months later.

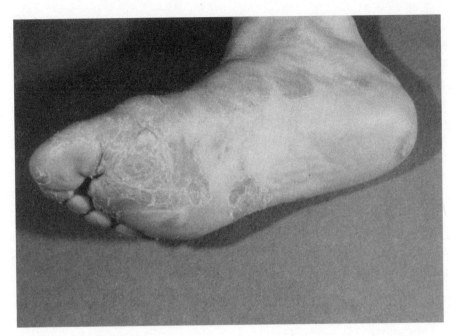

K.B., at the start of the regimen.

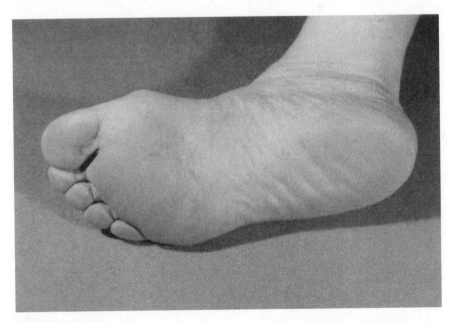

K.B., 10 months later.

One successful patient, having suffered from psoriasis for twenty years, was so pleased with the results obtained in the palms of his hands that he thought he could go out and chop wood. He did this for several hours. It took a few days, but the effect of that activity threw him into a spin—his hands flared up to a marked degree. He thought he was having a relapse, but it was nothing of the kind. I explained to him that it was a natural reaction to the localized abuse of his hands.

## Nail Psoriasis

One of the most unsightly features of the disease is when it appears on the fingernails and the toenails. It could get so thick under the nails (hyperkeratosis) that the nail bed lifts the nail right off its foundation. Yet I have seen complete regeneration of the nails and the surrounding structures take place. Admittedly, they take much longer to heal than lesions elsewhere on the body. It may take six months for a fingernail to regenerate and as much as a year or longer for toenails. Nevertheless, it can be done, and it has been done.

The procedure I worked out is clearly described in my cookbook, *Dr. John's Healing Psoriasis Cookbook . . . Plus!* To summarize, first be sure the condition is diagnosed by a dermatologist as psoriasis and is not a fungus, then:

1. Keep nails trimmed.
2. Follow the diet suggested herein.
3. Take one packet of Knox unflavored gelatin (or agar agar, in the case of vegetarians) per day, in water, juice, or anything that will make it palatable.
4. Take omega-3 fish oil or flaxseed oil supplements each day, as directed on the label.
5. Soak the hands (and the feet, if toes are also involved) in a large basin filled with comfortably hot water for fifteen to twenty minutes. (A small, portable whirlpool bath is preferred to a basin.)
6. Dry the hands and the feet (if involved) and vigorously apply any of the following throughout each nail: castor oil, olive oil–peanut oil mixture, emu oil, Bag Balm, Vaseline, Aquaphore, or

Aveeno lotion. Undoubtedly there are other products that can be effective, but these are the ones that I found work best.

7. Place a pair of white gym socks over the hands or the feet and retire for the night. This is to be done about four times per week, but no more.

I have seen time and again that following these relatively simply rules can bring about incredible results. There are three key words to practice: patience, patience, patience!

To reiterate, all other things being equal—that is, diet, spinal adjustments, enemas, and so forth—the best external treatment for people with psoriasis on the hands and the feet is hot soaks in an Epsom salts bath or a home whirlpool for about fifteen to twenty minutes, followed by thorough massages with peanut oil, castor oil, an olive oil–peanut oil mixture, cocoa butter, or coconut oil applied deeply into the hands or from the knees down in involvement of the feet. Plastic bags may be placed over the area being treated, followed by white gym socks, and left on for at least thirty minutes, often over-night. Lately, however, I am recommending that the plastic bags be omitted and the gym socks be used directly over the oils. This measure not only stops irritation but also prevents skin rot, which may possibly occur with those who are severely afflicted.

At first, these measures are carried out every night. After improve-ment takes place, treatment is cut back to three times per week, then to once a week, and is eventually eliminated altogether. In cases of pso-riatic arthritis, the hands and the feet are usually affected. The same treatment has proved equally beneficial in the vast majority of these cases but, invariably, more time is needed.

## A Lesson in Patience

An example of how patience eventually pays off is provided by one of my male patients who had psoriasis only on the palms of his hands. After suffering for fourteen years and being treated extensively by orthodox procedures without results, L.M. came to me as a last resort. In his case, it took fourteen months to clear his palms totally. This may seem like a long time to some, but he feels it was a small price to pay for a lifetime of freedom. "Fourteen months, after being afflicted

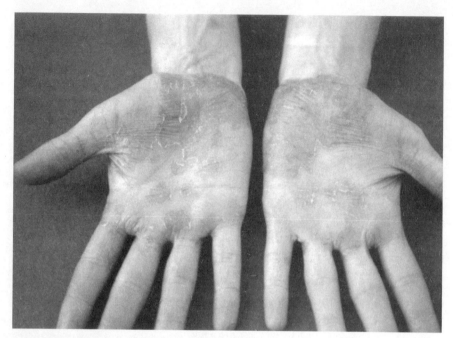

L.M., afflicted 14 years, at the start of the regimen.

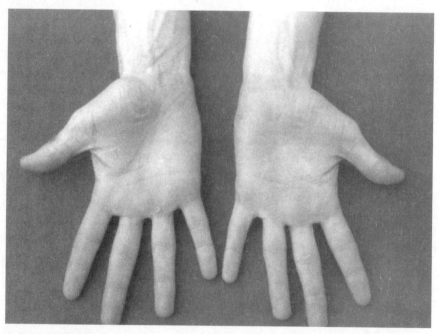

L.M., 14 months later.

fourteen years, isn't bad," according to L.M. After he cleared, I did not see him in my office again for five years. When he returned, it was for a back problem; his hands were still completely clear, even though he now cheats somewhat on his diet.

Although the procedures in this chapter deal primarily with external applications, diet was still the chief culprit in the cases discussed. It is interesting to mention that another patient of mine, who suffered with psoriasis on the palms of his hands, was practically addicted to Cajun (blackened) foods. He was improving quite nicely when on the prescribed diet, but one day, while dining out, the food he ordered was served Cajun style, which is prepared with hot spices. He was about to send it back but decided to try it anyway since he hadn't had it in such a long time. Although he enjoyed the meal, to his dismay the palms of his hands reacted almost immediately. He felt the sting in them within a few hours, convincing him that the hot spices somehow did, indeed, find their way to the palms of his hands.

What is the common denominator—in the cases presented in this chapter—among those who cleared up their psoriasis by following this alternate route when all else failed? Patience and persistence! In each of these cases, the patient fully recognized that he or she had exhausted all available therapies. In desperation, he or she followed the course I offered. Each was healed to his or her satisfaction, with everlasting joy and gratitude. Today, they are among my most helpful patients in convincing others to follow through with the regimen and to have faith. They are living examples of success achieved by believing that when you do the right thing, the right result will follow.

# CHAPTER 14

# The Healing Process

In an earlier chapter, I mentioned that one of my biggest problems in caring for psoriasis patients is holding their confidence until they actually see signs of true healing. Once this occurs, the patient is convinced that the process is working and that he or she is not wasting time, and he or she will usually follow through with greater enthusiasm.

Less itching, less scaling, and a general feeling of well-being are the first indications that the procedure is taking effect. There are visible signs that follow that act as proof-positive indications of healing; all psoriasis patients should learn to recognize these signs. I look upon them as types of healing that manifest in one of the following ways:

1. Healing becomes apparent from the start and continues to a successful outcome without drastic changes in the skin but with a slow, steady, gradual fading away of the lesions.

2. In circumscribed lesions, new skin begins to break through at the center of the lesion, giving a bull's-eye effect, and spreads to the outer edges (periphery) of the lesion, forming a rim, which, in time, also fades away. This type of clearing is observed best in the common vulgaris (plaque type) form of psoriasis.

3. The existing lesions spread out, join other lesions (coalesce), and appear as massive sheets of inflamed skin. The difference is that the diseased areas are now notably thinner, are less scaly, and gradually get lighter and lighter. New, regenerated skin begins to appear as a spotty effect, which widens until the

inflamed areas disappear, leaving the patient with a new skin surface. It is this third type of healing that we will primarily deal with in this chapter.

When I am sure that the patient followed the regimen faithfully, and such drastic changes occur as described in item 3, I conclude, without reservation, that he or she is truly on the road to recovery. It is only a matter of time before the apparent spreading flare-up will subside, for that type of reaction is part of the healing mechanism in that particular case. When the new skin breaks through and continues until all inflamed areas disappear, the joy of accomplishment on the part of the patient, as well as the physician, is indescribable.

## A Very Special Case

In early June 1990, the father of a beautiful seven-year-old called in a state of total desperation. Over the previous year, his young daughter, L.H., had developed a case of psoriasis. She had been diagnosed and treated by three dermatologists, without satisfactory results. Upon consulting with medical specialists at a leading psoriasis center in New York City, the father was informed that his daughter would have psoriasis all her life. The doctors recommended treatments with ultraviolet light administered at the hospital several times a week, as well as the application of cortisone creams. They left the hospital with a feeling of defeat. For the rest of their daughter's life, she would have to fight this terrible disease.

The day after the parents left the hospital, they heard of my work and immediately called me for a consultation. A more loving family could not be imagined. Their devotion and concern for one another struck me as the stuff dreams are made of.

We felt an instant rapport with one another. When I showed them the results I had obtained on a number of similar cases, their attitude instantly changed from total despair to possible hope. They all agreed to follow the regimen, especially the diet, and help little L.H. in any way they could.

At first L.H.'s skin seemed to react violently. Then, like magic, the psoriasis simply disappeared. It took a little over three months for L.H. to clear, with only the slightest spot or two remaining on her scalp.

Even these minor areas continued to fade with time. Her story is best told in the photographic sequence on pages 197–200.

This particular case stands out in my mind as one of the most profound, because I know L.H. did not deviate whatsoever from the regimen. Her devoted parents kept in touch with me constantly, assuring me that L.H. did not and would not stray from the program. As has happened with other cases in the past, when an initial flare-up took place and began to spread, coming together into solid sheets, L.H.'s parents became most concerned. It seemed everything was taking a turn for the worse. Drawing on past experience, my only advice was, "Keep going! Do not stop what you are doing." They agonized but reluctantly agreed. Soon the turning point came; new skin began to appear, and shortly thereafter the lesions faded away. The little girl's grateful father called to say, "It's just amazing! I can't believe it, the lesions are all gone!" A follow-up photo was taken one month later. The patient remains clear.

In the past, when some of my patients had such a reaction, they would quickly resort to orthodox methods to try to calm the skin down. I can understand this, but in doing so, they thwart the process and render this particular research invalid. In the case of L.H., however, it was the first time I ever had the opportunity to film the sequence without disruption or deviation from the regimen. Such a photographic progression has never been done before and should encourage others to continue with the procedure, knowing they are on the right track even when major flare-ups occur. Contrary to the assumption that the disease is running rampant and getting out of hand, despite appearances, it is a sign that the process is working.

Incidentally, the biggest dietary violation that I determined contributed to this girl's developing psoriasis was ketchup. Her mother informed me that her daughter had spread tomato ketchup on her bread practically every day for years. Once this practice stopped, combined with all other suggestions, the internal healing process began and continued to a successful conclusion.

Most important of all is the fact that this little girl was relieved of psoriasis at an early age, thereby warding off what very well could have been a lifetime of illness, discouragement, disfiguration, and untold expense for her parents. True, she probably will always have to be aware of her diet, but with such knowledge, she will also experience the greatest joy of all—that of never having to fear the disease again.

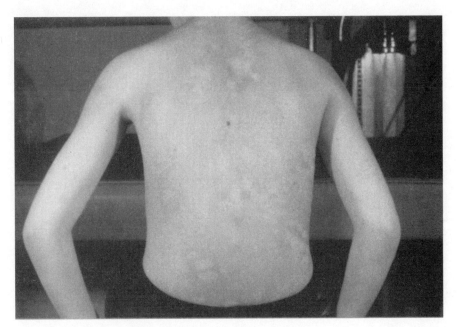

L.H. at the start of the regimen. The lesions are thick and scaly.

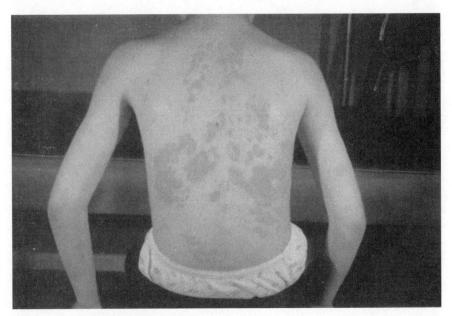

L.H. after 11 days; a generalized flare-up occurs.

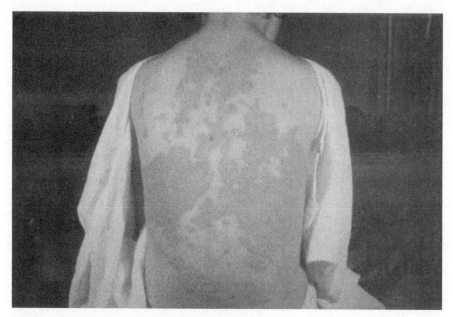

L.H. after 28 days. The lesions coalesce and become widespread, but there is less scaling, and the lesions are thinner with signs of new skin appearing.

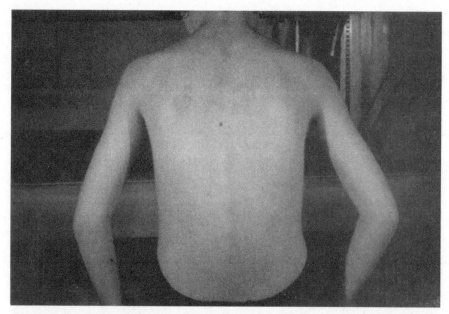

L.H. after 48 days. New skin replaces all inflamed areas, with only the slightest remains of previous lesions.

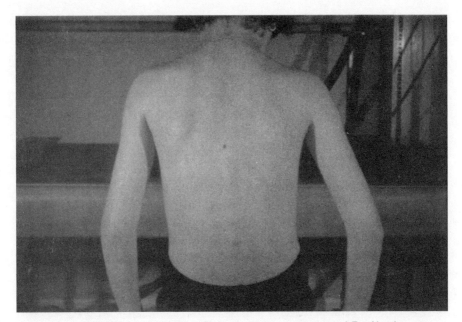

L.H. after 73 days. All lesions disappear. The entire torso is regenerated. Total healing time: 3 months, 1 week.

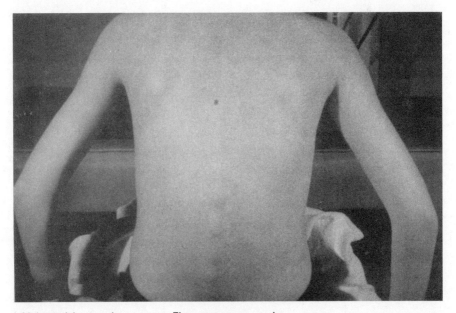

L.H. 1 month later, a close-up view. The patient remains clear.

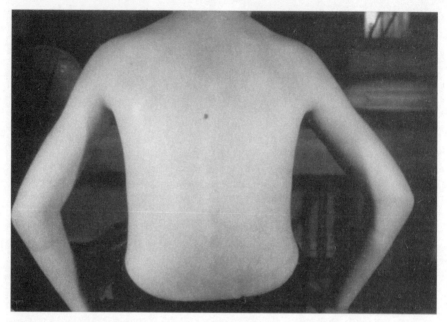

LH., taken 15 months later. Her skin is as smooth as silk.

Six years after the last photo was taken, L.H.'s parents reported to me that she was "just fine!" At times she had a spot or two pop up when she strayed from the diet, but it was nothing to speak of and was quickly brought under control.

# A Photographic Portfolio

The following photographic accounts represent a cross-section of some classic types of psoriasis cases treated successfully by following the Cayce/Pagano Natural Alternative approach to the disease. These patients followed through with patience and persistence, bringing about the desired end result.

# Case History

**Patient:** L.G. (female)

**Age:** 34

**Afflicted:** 22 years

**Diagnosis:** Psoriasis (generalized). Over 80 percent of her body was covered.

**Previous Management:** Extensive orthodox medical procedures for as long as she has had the disease.

**Results:** Within three months there was a marked improvement throughout her entire body. This progressive healing continued for the next two years. After clearing to her satisfaction, she remains in control of her condition.

**Remarks:** The basic regimen, combined with home enemas, played the major role in obtaining these results. This patient also admits that if she stopped smoking, she would have achieved results more rapidly.

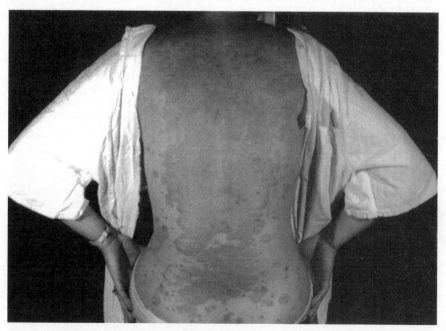

The patient before beginning the alternative regimen.

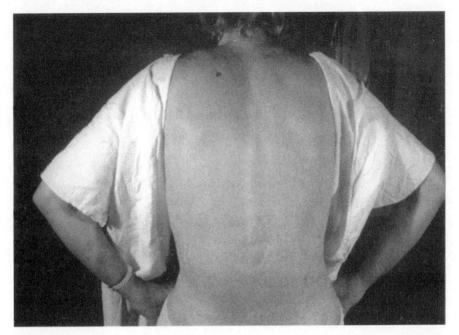

Three months later.

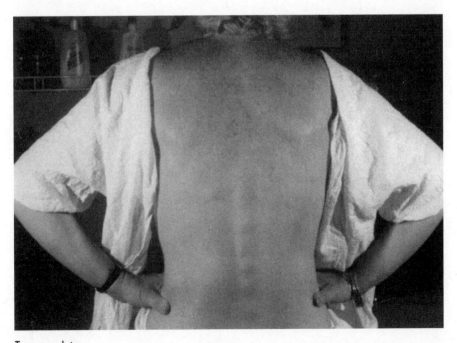

Two years later.

# Case History

**Patient:** J.C. (male)

**Age:** 30

**Afflicted:** 1 year

**Diagnosis:** Psoriasis (common/pustular).

**Previous Management:** Several medical procedures.

**Results:** Marked change in all lesions in two months; practically 100 percent clear in five months.

**Remarks:** This patient remained clear of all lesions for four years despite breaking his diet at times. When lesions began to reappear, he immediately went back on the regimen and brought it under control. Presently he is no longer plagued with the disease but he must be vigilant about his diet and eliminations.

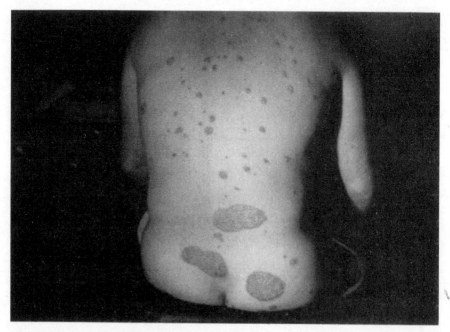

The patient before beginning the alternative regimen.

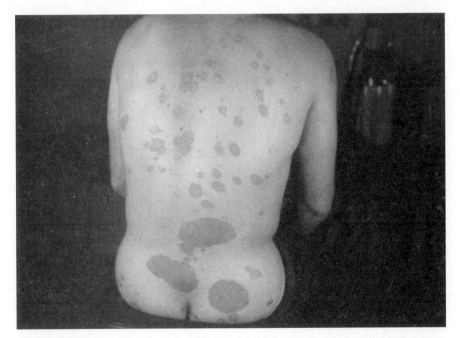

Two months later.

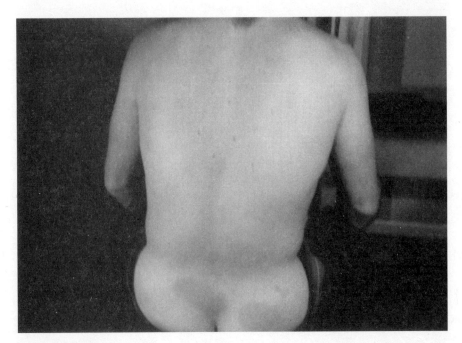

Five months later.

# Case History

**Patient:** J.R. (male)

**Age:** 36

**Afflicted:** 2 years

**Diagnosis:** Psoriasis (common vulgaris).

**Previous Management:** Under medical care—but not very extensive.

**Results:** Within four months, the lesions markedly improved. The patient was free of all lesions six months after starting the regimen but then reverted to his old dietary habits, and a lesion began to appear again on his left wrist. He learned that dietary control is most important.

**Remarks:** This patient was extremely overweight at the start of treatment. Within the year that it took to clear his psoriasis, he lost a total of sixty pounds. His figure transformed from total obesity to that of an athlete.

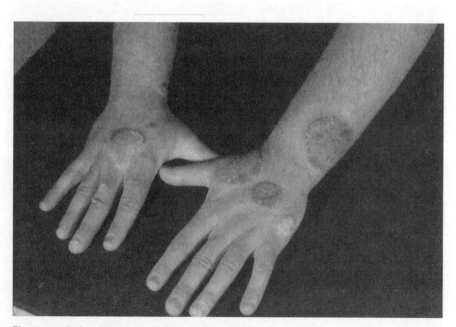

The patient before beginning the alternative regimen.

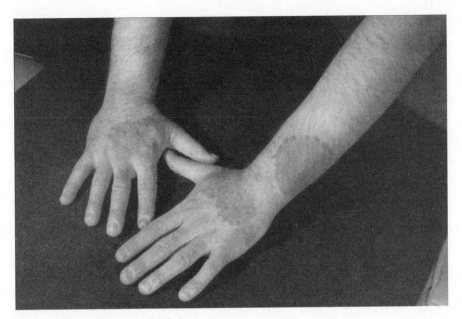

Four months later; lesions visibly fading.

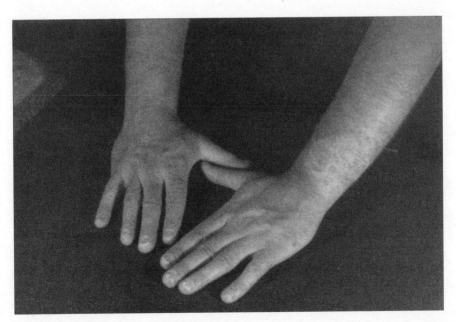

Thirteen months later.

# Case History

**Patient:** A.M. (female)

**Age:** 22

**Afflicted:** 6 years

**Diagnosis:** Psoriasis (generalized/erythrodermic). Over 90 percent of her body covered.

**Previous Management:** Extensive orthodox procedures—including hospitalization.

**Results:** Marked improvement in one month; almost 100 percent clear three months later.

**Remarks:** Diet played a significant role in healing this patient. Prior to her beginning the regimen, her diet consisted of pizza and chocolate practically every day.

*Note:* In this type of psoriasis, there is an overall redness of the skin surface—not unlike the shell of a boiled lobster. The only areas unaffected were the tips of the elbows.

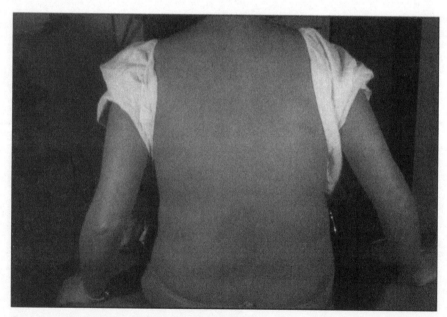

The patient before beginning the aternative regimen.

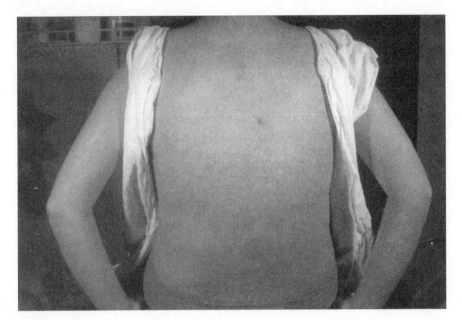

One month later.

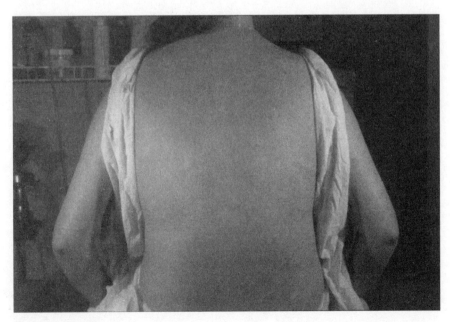

Three months later.

# Case History

**Patient**: M.F. (female)

**Age:** 22

**Afflicted:** 10 months

**Diagnosis:** Psoriasis (guttate)

**Previous Management:** The patient had been under the care of three dermatologists before beginning this regimen.

**Results:** The patient was completely clear of lesions four months after beginning.

**Remarks:** At first, results were slow. Rapid healing took place after the patient spent one week at the Association for Research and Enlightment for concentrated hydrotherapy and physiotherapy. When signs of recurrence began to appear due to straying from the diet for too long a period of time, resuming the regimen again brought the condition under control.

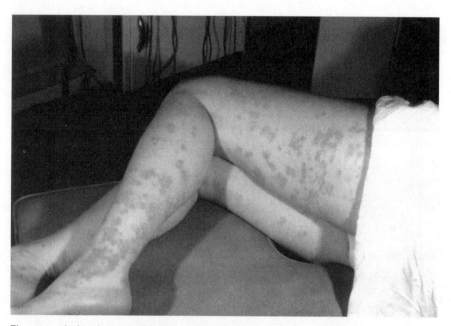

The patient before beginning the alternative regimen.

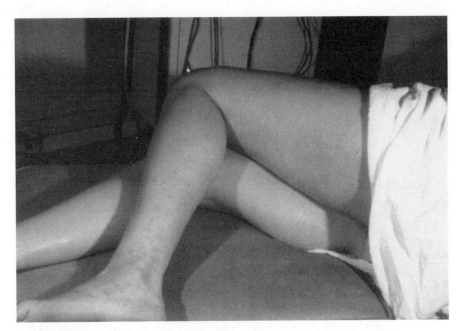

Two months later.

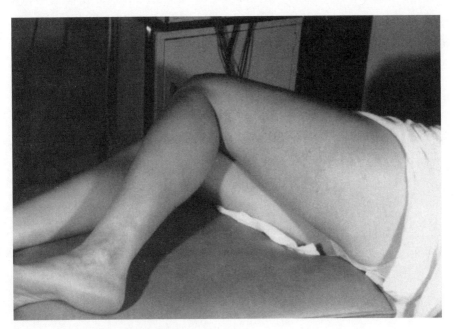

Four months later; clear of all lesions.

# Case History

**Patient:** T.O. (female)

**Age:** 14

**Afflicted:** 5 years

**Diagnosis:** Psoriasis (generalized). Over 75 percent of her body surface was covered with lesions.

**Previous Management:** Various orthodox medical procedures.

**Results:** Vast improvement in two months.

**Remarks:** This young girl was successful in her first attempt to follow this regimen. She had remained clear for over two years before lesions began to appear again and quickly spread through her entire skin surface. It was determined that the reason for this violent outbreak was her straying from the diet for too long a period of time by eating junk foods and eating too much of her favorite food—macaroni and cheese. Once she reverted back to the dietary rules of the regimen, spinal adjustments, proper eliminations, and the external application of hydrophilic ointment, her skin quickly responded. In two months, she was virtually clear of all lesions. She is in complete control of her condition.

*Note:* This patient healed so quickly that there was simply no time to take a photo of her at the midhealing stage; therefore, the only pictures shown are those of the initial stage, followed by the completed, healing stage of her abdomen and back.

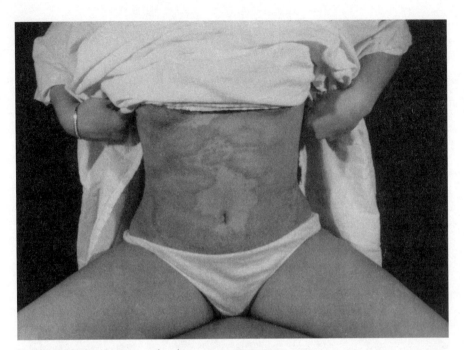

The patient before beginning the alternative regimen.

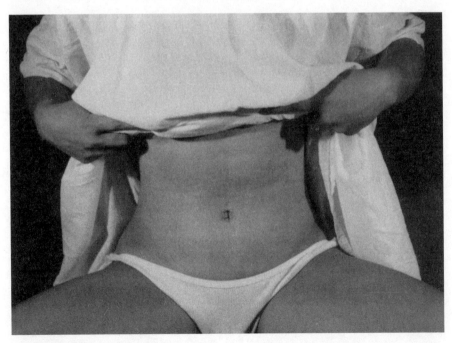

Two months later.

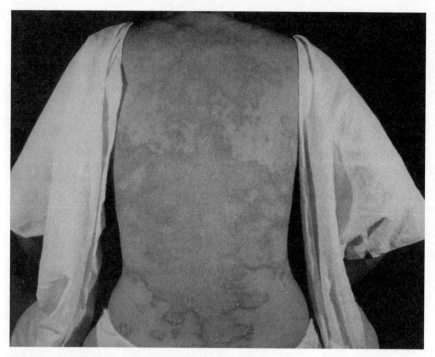

The patient before beginning the alternative regimen.

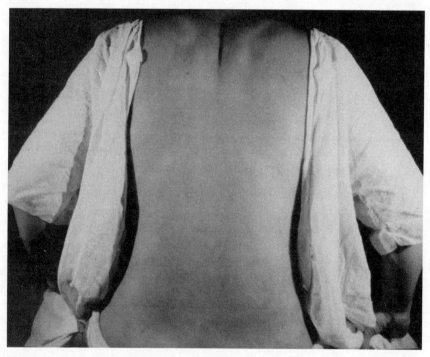

Two months later.

# CHAPTER 15

# Pushing the Panic Button

C rises arising from following this regimen have been very rare. In the past forty years or more, I cannot think of a single case where something occurred that put us in a spin. From experience, I've learned to alert my patients to certain changes (even if they are minor) that may occur while on the regimen, particularly in the first weeks. This warning usually takes care of any undue alarm, and the patient continues to follow through without concern.

There are, however, two reactions in particular that understandably disturb some patients, regardless of my warnings.

1. New lesions may erupt in different areas, making it appear that the disease is spreading (such as in the case of little L.H., as depicted in chapter 14).

2. A weight loss (sometimes considerable) may occur, but this is usually desirable.

These two reactions, if they occur, are the most troublesome to deal with. My advice is:

1. Ignore the new lesions and carry on with the regimen. In every case to date, the new lesions eventually faded and disappeared.

2. In the case of weight loss (if it bothers you), "double up" on the food you are permitted to consume but don't go overboard. Hunger should never be a problem, but remember, eating too much of even the permitted foods can cause an overtaxation of the digestive process. Moderation is still the key.

## Family Reactions

A family member's reaction can be as troublesome as a patient's. If, for instance, a child or a spouse is not responding 100 percent from the very beginning, a family member may overreact and thereby discourage the patient.

One young patient, rather severely afflicted with psoriasis, followed all instructions in taking his Epsom salts bath. Immediately upon completion of the bath, while the pores of his skin were naturally wide open, he covered himself with Cuticura ointment (not the right time for this ointment to be used). His body became inflamed. His mother, in a panic, called and demanded an explanation. What should she do? He was "burning up." After the terror subsided and the accusations ceased, I was able to explain to her what the boy had done. Instead of using the olive oil–peanut oil combination, which is called for after an Epsom salts bath, he had used the acidic Cuticura ointment all over his body. Obviously, his skin reacted violently. The remedy was simple: to shower away the ointment from the skin. He did and was immediately relieved.

Here was a clear case of familial overreaction, although an understandable one. This does not imply that all families will react emotionally in the same way.

You may recall that one of my youngest patients in the early years of my experimentation was A.S. At the time, I had no explanation for why new lesions were forming where they had never been before. Both parent and patient had followed the rules of the regimen religiously. "That's all right, Dr. Pagano," his mother said. "We said we would give you three months and we will stick to it." Stick to it they did. In time, not only the old, but the new lesions had faded away. As A.S.'s mother remarked, one day they looked, and the lesions were simply not there.

From this early experience, I learned and taught my patients to follow through with the regimen without being in a hurry. You cannot set a time limit for the disappearance of the lesions. Those patients who were successful simply did what was required of them without fuss or bother and allowed nature to take its course.

## When Prompt Attention Is Necessary

Two young, attractive women, who had suffered with psoriasis for many years, began therapy at the same time. They were eager to see the process in action. One even began to show signs of improvement within the first week, especially behind her ears. The other did not show any appreciable change, but there was a marked improvement in her eliminations.

After the third week, however, their enthusiasm changed to discouragement. The girl who was so pleased with the healing behind her ears was deeply upset because lesions now broke out all over her face, particularly on her forehead. It looked very much like prickly heat, but, of course, it was not. The other girl was distressed due to inflamed areas in her genital region. The pruritus (itching) became unbearable, keeping her up all hours of the night. Nothing seemed to help. She reported she was doing well on the diet and other measures, if only it were not for the itching.

For the patient with new lesions on her face, I advised her to brew a pot of saffron tea, place a towel over her head and the teapot, and allow the tea's gentle vapors (not too hot) to suffuse her face. After repeating this treatment over two days, the lesions began to disappear. By the following week, they were practically gone, and her eagerness to continue treatment was renewed.

For the other young lady, I recommended a sitz bath with about one-third to one-half bottle of Glyco-Thymoline mixed in the water. This gave her the first sense of relief in weeks. Later she had only to pat Glyco-Thymoline, full strength, on severely affected areas, and the relief was almost immediate. A good substitute for Glyco-Thymoline could be the ever-popular Lavoris.

In both cases, as in others, it was important that quick adjustments in treatment be made before the patient lost faith in the procedure.

## Allergic Reactions

Anyone can develop an allergy. It is very important that your allergy history be established before any treatment is undertaken. Allergic reactions can occur to anything from a blade of grass to a strand of hair, not only to foods or medications. Usually the existence of an allergic reaction is established only *after* it has taken place. Even allergy testing beforehand is not foolproof, nor is it completely accurate in its evaluation. The rule regarding allergies is simple: Once an allergen has been determined, it is best to stay away from it.

Physical reactions manifest in a number of ways, such as skin rash or swelling and irritation of mucus membranes. Asthmatic attacks as well as changes in mood or mentality (such as violent behavior, aggression, or confusion) can also be attributed to allergens. Reactions can vary from a minor annoyance to incapacitation requiring hospitalization. Regardless of the degree experienced, an allergy of any kind should not be taken lightly, and any necessary measure should be taken to counteract or avoid triggering it.

A dear friend and patient of mine cannot have the tiniest piece of a pecan. If she does it could mean a matter of life or death. Her throat constricts, cutting off her air passage. Hospitalization and adrenaline shots are necessary to counteract the allergic reaction. Similar incidents are common with some people when they consume shellfish or peanuts. The list of allergens seems endless. In many severe cases, "pushing the panic button" is justified.

Although allergic reactions resulting from the dietary measures outlined in this book are rare, they do, at times, occur in some people. The individual must take responsibility for determining which foods he is allergic to.

For instance, broccoli is a highly desirable vegetable and encouraged as part of the diet. Yet one of my patients has a severe digestive disturbance and skin flare-up when she consumes the smallest amount of it. Carrots are to be eaten as often as possible, perhaps as frequently as lettuce and celery. You may recall, however, that I had one patient who could *eat* them without experiencing any problems as long as she did not *touch* them. Upon touching them, her fingers would become inflamed immediately. Another patient cannot even bring a raw apple to her mouth. If she does, her lips swell up like balloons. These reactions, although relatively rare, must be recognized and respected. If a patient finds that he or she is supersensitive to any of the measures called for in this regimen, my advice is clear: avoid them!

Substitutes can always be found for practically every measure. With a little time, patience, and observation, one can reach a workable alternative that will help avoid future undesirable episodes.

## The Terrible Time: Herxheimer Reaction

Invariably, when the purge period, the healing crisis, the inflammatory stage, or what I call "the storm before the calm" takes place, you will understandably cry out for relief. A flare-up occurs with incredible inflammation, dryness, and tautness of the skin, to the extent that you can hardly move or take a deep breath. You may stay in bed for days because the thought of moving is unbearable. In most cases you are experiencing dehydration. Water ingested, as well as applied externally, may help considerably. At times, hospitalization may be necessary for intravenous feeding. You must keep the internal environment of the body cells, as well as the epidermis (surface layer of the skin), as moist as possible. Cracked lips and dryness of the skin to the point of pain on the slightest movement may occur. Even light clothing or bed sheets touching the skin may be intolerable. It is during this period, the "terrible time," that the patient and the doctor must have faith in the process and realize that the body is "doing its thing" and purging the system of all toxic elements.

The Herxheimer Reaction was named after the doctor who first recognized it. Know it for what it is: the body is throwing off toxins, called the die-off period. It is the precursor to eventual healing of the skin.

Do whatever is necessary to make yourself comfortable. Applying warm damp cloths to the hottest parts of the body and allowing them to cool on the skin, or sitting in a tub of tepid water to keep the skin as moist as possible, will give temporary relief. Scaling is usually profuse, and oozing pus occurs in the most severe cases (pustular psoriasis). Again, hospitalization may be necessary. Enemas, or even a high colonic, can be very helpful immediately. Alka-Seltzer, or any antacid product, will also help calm the skin down. If anti-inflammatory medication is called for, you should take it, as prescribed by your physician. Nevertheless, I have seen these periods of sheer torture gradually subside in a few days, with less itching and flattening and smoothing of the skin. Most important of all is the appearance of new skin areas beginning to show through. When this occurs, you are on the road to recovery. This is not to say there will not be further flare-ups; in fact, there usually are. However, they are not as severe as before. When my patients adhere to the regimen, I have rarely failed to see it deliver. Time and patience are paramount. Give the body a chance to purge itself; you will be glad you did.

## Cooling the Flames

I have used three simple but effective methods that help calm and cool the skin in severe flare-ups. To repeat, it is very helpful to take a home enema or a high colonic irrigation, if practical. This, in itself, can spell the difference between constant suffering and immediate relief.

After the enema or the colonic, one of the following often proves successful:

1. *Hot bed sheet application (assistance required).* A large plastic sheet is placed on the bed with a lightweight blanket on top. The patient strips down and lies on the blanket. In the meantime, a bedsheet is soaking in comfortably hot water. When the patient is positioned on the bed, the hot, but not scalding, bedsheet is wrung out and placed over the patient (with the head exposed, of course) and tucked into all contours of the body. The hot sheet will not be a shock to the system, since the skin is already inflamed. The patient simply lies there while the sheet begins to cool down. As this cooling occurs, it is pulling the inflammation out of the body, offering considerable relief to the patient. The patient may then turn over and repeat the process on the other side. It may require two or three applications a day until the inflammation completely subsides. A good moisturizer is applied between each application while the skin is still wet.

2. *The pajama shower.* The patient puts on a pair of cotton pajamas and steps into a warm to hot shower and soaks down. The water is turned off and the patient remains standing in the shower stall until the pajamas begin to cool. This will rather quickly cool down the surface of the body, even to the point that the patient's teeth may chatter. The pajamas are then removed and

a moisturizer applied over the wet skin. This may be repeated every two hours until a certain degree of comfort is experienced. The patient then puts on a dry pair of pajamas and retires for the night.

3. *The pajama bath.* The bathtub is filled with comfortably hot water, and the patient, wearing cotton pajamas, gets into the tub. Once the pajamas are saturated, the drain is opened and the water is allowed to run out. The patient remains in the tub until the pajamas start to cool down and he or she feels the chilling effect. The patient then gets out of the tub, removes the pajamas, and, while he or she is still wet, applies a moisturizer. Then the patient puts on dry pajamas and retires for the night. This procedure may be repeated as often as deemed necessary.

These are the procedures used at times in hospitals when a patient suffers the Herxheimer Reaction. This reaction is not to be prevented; it is to be controlled by whatever means available. The important thing is to prevent dehydration. Therefore, drinking pure water and providing moist applications to the skin surface are the rules of the day. They are the only way water is induced into the body, unless intravenous feeding is called for in a hospital setting. Tepid water enemas can also help prevent dehydration.

# CHAPTER 16

# The Arthritic Connection: Psoriatic Arthritis

Among the millions of psoriatics, a small but significant number suffer with a double jeopardy—psoriasis combined with arthritis. Although the clinical features resemble other forms of arthritis, particularly rheumatoid, serological tests have a positive rheumatoid factor in rheumatoid arthritis but not necessarily in psoriatic arthritis.

Experts cannot agree on the correlation between the incidence of psoriasis and arthritis. According to a study by the researcher Gibble, 2.5 to 5.5 percent of rheumatoid arthritis patients have psoriasis. Broad range estimates vary from less than 1 percent to 32 percent, presumably owing to the various definitions of arthritis. Figures aside, the fact remains that the combination of the two problems, on the skin and in the joints, can create havoc with the individual and can, in the severe cases, lead to invalidism. Fortunately, these cases number relatively few among psoriatics, but they do occur, and I have seen my fair share of them.

Psoriatic arthritis requires more work, patience, and discipline than any other form of psoriasis. For one thing, the person probably began this disease process many years before starting treatment. It has been estimated that some patients have had skin lesions for twenty or thirty years before they started experiencing joint disease.

Psoriatic arthritis has been recognized for about a hundred years, and even in this form, there are different classifications. For instance, there is *asymmetric oligoarthritis,* which affects the majority of psoriatic arthritics (70 percent). *Oligo* refers to "few" or "little" joints, especially those in the hands near the knuckles. Then there is *symmetric polyarthritis,* which closely resembles rheumatoid arthritis, but a blood test does not show a positive rheumatoid factor. This constitutes about 15 percent of those afflicted. *Polyarthritis* is a third form (about 5 percent) in which many joints are affected, usually near the fingertips and also in the feet. This type is considered the classic type of psoriatic arthritis. A fourth type is *psoriatic spondylitis* (also about 5 percent). In psoriatic spondylitis, the vertebrae are involved, to a greater or lesser degree, and should be of prime interest to the chiropractor or osteopath. (Look for more on this later on in this chapter, in the section titled "Poker Spine.") The fifth type is *arthritis mutilans.* Again, only 5 percent of psoriatic arthritics are affected by it, but it is the most destructive type. In this type there is bone destruction and deformity.

## About Arthritis

Arthritis can strike anyone; it is no respecter of age. Its proportions range from minor aches and pains to complete incapacitation. Unless the cause is related directly to trauma or infection, its origin is largely unknown, but the one certainty common to most forms is inflamed joints.

The word *arthritis* is derived from the Greek prefix *arthron,* meaning "pertaining to a joint," and the Greek suffix *itis,* meaning "inflammation." There are about a hundred forms of the disease, but the most common forms by far are rheumatoid arthritis (RA) and osteoarthritis (DJD—degenerative joint disease).

Approximately 36 million Americans are afflicted with arthritis, with a million new cases occurring each year. Over 7 million arthritics have some disability, and about 3 million are seriously impaired. There are 8 million people crippled with RA. Estimates show that three times more women than men contract this most serious form, even in childhood. Although the explanation for this discrimination is unknown, researchers are now questioning hormonal factors. Psoriatic arthritis, however, is found equally in men and women.

## Is There a Virus Link?

A March 24, 1984, *New York Daily News* article by Judith Randal, "Link a Virus to Arthritis," related that scientists have succeeded in isolating a virus—the RA-1 virus—that may cause rheumatoid arthritis. Dr. Robert Simpson of the Waksman Institute of Microbiology at Rutgers University feels this discovery may eventually lead to more effective treatment of the disease and possibly to a preventive vaccine. He also said that his findings may make it possible to discover the cause of other diseases related to rheumatoid arthritis.

Since some features of psoriatic arthritis closely resemble those of rheumatoid arthritis (such as morning stiffness, pain on motion, tenderness, and swelling of small joints of the hands and the feet), it behooves us to review some interesting Cayce concepts.

## Same Problem, Different View

At first glance, it would appear that the aforementioned concept of viral invasion is worlds apart from the Cayce theory. A closer look, however, reveals that they are not so far apart; they just differ in their basic premise.

Although viruses, bacteria, and airborne and interior destructive elements surround us, most of them are rendered harmless in the healthy body. It is when the healthy body breaks down in some fashion that these destructive elements take over. Cayce claims that in arthritis, particularly rheumatoid, a high acidic nature of the body permits the virus or some other organism to thrive. It could be that the researchers at Rutgers University have isolated a virus relative to rheumatoid arthritis. Questions remain, however: Would this virus thrive in a different environment, that is, one that is alkaline rather than acidic? Should efforts be centered on destroying the virus, or should they be concentrated on changing the internal environment of the host, that is, the body chemistry of the patient?

According to Cayce, maintaining alkalinity in the body, primarily through diet, will render a person virtually immune to such congestions. He particularly singled out *lettuce, carrots,* and *celery* as the most effective foods that help render the body alkaline.

If this is true, it follows that changing one's chemical, internal environment to alkaline is beneficial in warding off, preventing, or alleviating many arthritic conditions. Since this can be done primarily through diet and other safe methods, the research would not be expensive or invasive. Some of my patients have done it on their own with excellent results. True, Cayce did not identify a specific virus, as did Dr. Simpson and his associates at Rutgers. Nevertheless, Cayce's theory is not easily shrugged off when one considers the findings of Dr. Charles P. Lucas of the Wayne State University School of Medicine.

According to Dr. Lucas, who is also chief of endocrinology and metabolism at Harper-Grace Hospitals, debilitating pain and severe joint swelling stemming from rheumatoid arthritis can be virtually eliminated when sufferers switch to a strict low-fat diet. A February 10, 1982, Associated Press article titled, "Low-Fat Diet Said to Ease Arthritis," quoted Dr. Lucas at a Detroit press conference: "I can't say that the low-fat diet is a cure, because as soon as patients go off that diet, their arthritis returns. But they can stay almost completely free of symptoms by eliminating fats from their diets."

Patients on the diet Dr. Lucas speaks of are allowed to eat whole wheat bread and cereals, vegetables, fruits, skim milk, rice, macaroni, and gelatin, among other foods, but they are not allowed any meats and can eat only saltwater fish. Except for one or two minor items, one would think his diet came right out of the Cayce archives. If Cayce stressed anything about arthritis or psoriasis, it was to eliminate fats and eat many fresh fruits and vegetables.

The psoriatic arthritic must also be very careful to avoid salt and salted products in particular. Just a pat of salted butter can flare up swollen ankles or wrists to a marked degree. When one of my patients substituted a little sweet butter for salted butter, she immediately experienced a difference. She then took the time to read labels and avoided salted products as much as possible. In her particular case, the swelling of the ankles and the wrists diminished in a matter of days, walking was much easier, and generalized aches and pains subsided to an appreciable degree.

This same patient substituted skim milk for whole milk, because whole milk contains salt as well as fat. Ice cream also has salt and fat in it, so she ate yogurt. She selected low-fat, low-salt, or no-salt cheeses. Her body was becoming her servant, rather than the other way around.

Why? Because she took the time to study her own reactions, she read labels, and she became creative in solving her own problems.

Further research on the effects certain foods have on arthritis is revealed in the works of Dr. Norman F. Childers of the University of Florida and founder of the Nightshades Research Foundation. As stated earlier, Childers has traced the adverse affects the nightshade family of plants has on the arthritic. His prescription is the No-Nightshade Diet. His research is gaining in popularity with patients as well as physicians.

If one were to combine the findings of Dr. Lucas and Dr. Childers and add a touch of Cayce, a formula evolves to ward off arthritis as well as psoriasis: Eliminate fats, the nightshades, sweets, and alcohol. Drink plenty of fresh water. Eat large quantities of fresh fruits and select vegetables. Fish, fowl, and lamb are permitted, but nothing fried. (Cayce is more lenient than the researchers are, in that he allows fowl and lamb.) Nevertheless, in the vast majority of cases, given adequate time, this regimen works.

## A Picture Evolves

The discourses of Edgar Cayce never included a file under the heading "psoriatic arthritis." However, extensive treatises on the individual conditions psoriasis and arthritis are available. As a matter of fact, these two conditions are among the top ten circulating files most frequently requested by the over twenty thousand members of the Cayce Foundation.

Careful study of the two files reveals a close similarity in managing both of these conditions. Common sense dictates that a combination of the therapeutic regimens for psoriasis and rheumatoid arthritis is the best and most reasonable course to follow. My advice to my patients with psoriatic arthritis is:

1. Follow the psoriasis regimen to the letter.
2. Add the following measures derived from the discourses on rheumatoid arthritis.
   - Have a full-body peanut-oil massage twice a week, if possible. Leave the oil on for at least a half hour or overnight

after the massage before washing it off. Shower down, but do not use soap.

- Take a peanut-oil tub bath. To a tub of comfortably hot water, add one cup of cold-pressed peanut oil. Submerge up to the neck and remain in the water at least a half hour. As the water cools, add additional hot water. (*Caution:* Peanut-oil baths leave the tub very slippery. The patient *must* be sure to have help getting into and out of the tub. After the bath, the patient pats himself dry, leaving the light coating of peanut oil on overnight. Clearly it's best to do this just before bedtime.)

- Add Jerusalem artichokes (sunchokes) to the diet, once a week.

- Avoid bananas and strawberries and too many fruits in general.

- Eat all kinds of raw vegetables (except cabbage, which can cause constipation) in Knox gelatin. These may include watercress, chard, mustard greens, kale, carrots, celery, and lettuce (leaf or romaine). These vegetables must be prepared within the gelatin—as a gelatin salad. As mentioned in chapter 6, gelatin has been called a catalyst in the body, helping it to better absorb the vitamins and other nutrients of fruits and vegetables.

- Cleanse the colon by using high colonic irrigations or high enemas, as these play a significant role in alleviating arthritis. Colonics or high enemas should be used approximately every ten days, from the beginning of therapy, for at least two months. Thereafter, once a month until all symptoms subside, then about four times a year, at the change of seasons. This pattern may vary with individual patients.

- Avoid alcoholic drinks.

Since rheumatoid arthritis is so closely tied to psoriatic arthritis, the same precautionary measures apply. Do not disturb the body too greatly, and expect the regimen to take more time. The course to follow in psoriatic arthritic cases is the slow, gentle approach.

The above measures are those that I found most practical. A most informative treatise on both arthritis and psoriasis is found in the *Physician's Reference Notebook,* compiled and edited by William A. McGarey, MD, the director of the Medical Research Division of the Association for Research and Enlightenment (ARE) and published by the ARE Press. This volume, once available only to licensed physicians, is now available to the public through the ARE bookstore.

## Avoiding "Winter Itch" (Asteatotic Dermatitis)

The psoriatic arthritic patients I have encountered seem to be more affected by the itch, with tightening and cracking of the skin, in winter months than do the patients who have only psoriasis to contend with. This is due to the lack of moisture in the skin and is caused by the dry environment in the household that occurs when turning on the heat.

Three of the best remedies for this problem are mentioned in chapter 9, under the heading "Physiotherapy at Home." They are the whirlpool, the humidifier, and drinking plenty of fresh water. A home whirlpool treatment, using comfortably hot water for approximately twenty minutes, followed by a gentle peanut-oil massage, will not only feel comforting but will also help retain moisture in the skin.

In winter, Epsom salts baths are generally to be avoided, as they tend to dry out the skin too much. I do advise, however, to add one-half to one cup of peanut oil to the water while the whirlpool is operating. After the prescribed amount of time, the patient carefully emerges from the tub, pats the skin dry, and relaxes. (People must remember to observe the necessary precautions. They must not use a whirlpool if they suffer from a heart condition of any kind. They must make certain that there is someone on hand in the unlikely event of a fainting spell and also to assist them in getting into and out of the tub.)

A humidifier is extremely helpful in keeping the air in the room moist, especially while you are sleeping. Breathing in moist air helps avoid the drawing of moisture from the skin and allows the surface cells to remain pliable. Thorough cleansing of these units daily is essential to prevent spores from forming that may become airborne, potentially causing respiratory ailments. Many excellent brands now have filters to help prevent spores from being distributed. Instructions are provided by the manufacturer. Still, to be on the safe side, clean them periodically.

Again, both portable home whirlpools and humidifiers are available in department stores at a nominal cost. I consider them a wise investment for the psoriatic arthritic.

## Stress and Its Effects

Since the cause of arthritis is unknown and the cause of psoriasis is unknown (from the orthodox point of view), it follows that the cause of psoriatic arthritis is likewise unknown. I am often prone to follow a simple rule in trying to get to the bottom of a patient's condition: ask the patient! In my opinion, every physician should ask his patient, "What do you think is the cause of your condition?" Some of the answers are amazing, and it is even more astonishing to see how accurate the patient can be when a diagnosis is finally reached.

Based on the patients I have seen throughout the years, it seems to me that in the case of psoriatic arthritis, stressful living conditions heads the list of possible basic causes.

I have had a good number of severely afflicted straight psoriasis or straight arthritic cases who lived under ideal conditions (at least by outward appearance). On the other hand, I have rarely, if ever, found a psoriatic arthritic case whose living conditions were ideal. Of course, the question "Which came first—the chicken or the egg?" may be asked. In other words, did the stressful living conditions cause the illness, or did the illness bring about stressful living conditions? Regardless of which came first, there was a slow but steady buildup of toxins in the body before the victim found that he or she could not get out of bed one morning.

I believe that negative attitudes and emotions play a significant role in these cases, creating stress, tension, and anxiety and all that goes with it, even though the person may feel some justification in harboring such attitudes.

Anger, for instance, is only one of the negative states of mind that lends itself to creating a stressful atmosphere. Other contributing emotions are fear, jealousy, loneliness, insecurity (financial or otherwise), job pressure (actual or imaginary), inharmonious family life, and other similar situations, all of which can yield the same result: a sick body formed by a sick soul.

# Atomodine

No account of the Edgar Cayce approach to arthritis, particularly the rheumatoid type, would be complete without mentioning a substance called Atomodine (atomic iodine). It is called for in several systemic conditions, especially in the long-standing, degenerative-type diseases like psoriatic arthritis. Atomodine is valuable because it is iodine in a form apparently less toxic to the body than the molecular iodine generally available in kelp tablets or Lugol's Solution.

As a chiropractic physician, I cannot personally prescribe the use of Atomodine, for to do so borders on practicing medicine. I only mention the substance's existence for those readers and researchers who might not have heard of it before. In such cases, I therefore advise my patients to first consult with a medical doctor or osteopath regarding the use of Atomodine. (*Caution:* Under no circumstances should Atomodine be used without medical approval.) One drop of it supplies about six times the minimum daily requirement of iodine, and too much iodine can lead to overstimulation of the thyroid gland, resulting in nervousness, insomnia, and rapid heartbeat. A person allergic to even the smallest amount of iodine can have a severe reaction. Nevertheless, approximately 610 Cayce readings enthusiastically mention Atomodine in cases involving glandular deficiency or malfunction associated with a shortage of iodine in the system. Atomodine was rarely prescribed as a treatment by itself but was to be used as a part of various programs involving other important measures.

One of the many recommendations for its use is to take it internally for cases of arthritis. Its purpose is to "purify" the glands, and the recommended dosage is only one drop of Atomodine in half a glass of water a few days out of the week, then skipping it for about a week, then beginning again. Different patients were offered different suggestions on how much to take. That is why the substance must not be used indiscriminately. I found it quite interesting to discover some readings stating that for greatest effectiveness, spinal adjustments are to be given in conjunction with the taking of Atomodine.

## Glyco-Thymoline

Keep in mind that the underlying common denominator for the psoriatic arthritic is to reduce acidity and promote alkalinity of the body. The use of the substance Glyco-Thymoline taken internally (just a few drops in a glass of water) holds an honored place when it comes to internal purification, as does Atomodine.

Glyco-Thymoline, a mouthwash, is useful to the psoriatic not only when taken internally to cleanse and purify the intestinal tract, but also when used externally, as an antipruritic (itch reducer). Applied full strength to the irritated areas, it often works when all else fails. Since itching is a major problem for some, it is helpful to keep a bottle of the alkaline formula handy. A very effective and simple method of use is to put a 50/50 mixture of water and Glyco-Thymoline in a spray bottle and spray it on areas that itch.

Therefore, there are only three substances within the Edgar Cayce regimen for psoriasis and/or arthritis that should be first approved by a medical doctor or an osteopath. They are: Atomodine, Glyco-Thymoline, and the tri-salts compound (sulfur, cream of tartar, and Rochelle salts), which we covered in chapter 5. Although they are nonprescription items and may be obtained from the Cayce product suppliers (see appendix D), since they are to be taken internally, they should be approved by practitioners licensed in dispensing drugs.

## Swollen Joints

When the joints of the body become severely swollen and inflamed, the psoriatic arthritic becomes practically incapacitated. The pain can be excruciating, movement extremely limited, and weight bearing next to impossible. It is obviously most devastating when the ankles are affected, because of the restrictions this places on mobility.

Any joint or number of joints can be affected: ankles, small bones of the feet, knees, hip joints, shoulders, wrists, and small bones of the hand. A very effective treatment is outlined in chapter 13. In the case of psoriatic arthritis of these areas, the therapy is similar.

All things being equal, that is, diet, colonics or enemas, water intake, and so forth, the use of hot soaks in Epsom salts baths followed by peanut-oil joint massage has been found to be extremely helpful. Sufferers are advised to make a hot Epsom salts solution by adding one-half to one pound of the salts to a basin or bowl three-quarters full of hot water. If the hands are being treated, the hands and wrists should be soaked in the water for five minutes, working the wrists in various directions. The hands should be massaged together while working the fingers and rotating the joints, then the patient should continue soaking for another five or ten minutes. Next the patient should pat dry the hands. At this point, 100 percent pure cold-pressed peanut oil should be rubbed into the hands, the wrists, and up the arms. Then disposable plastic or plain cotton gloves, which can be purchased at any discount beauty supply shop or drugstore, should be worn. The gloves are left on for at least an hour, or even overnight. This same basic procedure is used for the ankles and the feet, but a large plastic bag is used in place of gloves and covered with white socks. Many have reported using a bag and a white sock for each hand as well, in place of gloves, and many use only a white sock without the bag. Whatever is more comfortable should be used. A knee-high gym sock can cover the entire hand, wrist, and forearm up to the elbow, which often has visible lesions.

If you have a small whirlpool designed for the hands and the feet, such as the Oster, I recommend it be used every other day. Some peanut oil can be placed in the water of the massage unit. After use, there may be a problem lifting up the unit to empty out the water. If there is no one handy to lift up the unit, it can be emptied simply by using a quart-size container to remove the water bucket by bucket. Although this may be a little awkward, it is better than not using the unit at all.

Hot Epsom salts packs are also very helpful for swollen joints. They are made by soaking a small terry cloth towel in hot water that has been saturated with Epsom salts. You can tell that the water is saturated with Epson salts when the salts no longer dissolve but remain visible at the bottom of the basin. After squeezing excess water out of the towel, wrap it around the joint being treated and cover it with plastic wrap. An electric (waterproof) heating pad is then placed around the entire setup. In cases involving the wrist, the knees, the elbows, or the ankles, the Gillette wraparound electric heat unit, or something similar, is most effective.

I advise my patients to leave the heating pad on low or medium heat for about twenty minutes, or whatever seems comfortable to them. When they remove the heating unit, they are to massage peanut oil into the joint. At times, I have recommended rubbing warm peanut oil on the joint first, then placing the Epsom salts pack over it followed by the heating pad. Admittedly, this is a bit of a bother, but once the routine is established, it becomes second nature—especially when the patient begins to feel better.

It must not be assumed that the coexistence of psoriatic lesions and joint pain automatically labels the diagnosis psoriatic arthritis. It may be a simultaneous condition of gout, rheumatoid arthritis, or even systemic lupus erythematosus (LE). In these less-typical cases, serological tests for the rheumatoid factor, and an LE cell preparation, should be made medically, which may assist in establishing a diagnosis.

From an X-ray point of view, the most striking histopathologic alteration in psoriatic arthritis is the destructive bone changes near the joint surface and in the adjacent shaft. An X-ray of the small joints of the hands and the feet is often helpful in evaluating the extent of the disease. The radiologist will look for signs of erosion of osseous (bone) tissue, particularly in the distal phalangeal joints (fingertips), as well as destruction of bone in the metatarsal and interphalangeal joints of the feet.

These are all clinical findings and are really the concern of the diagnostician. The point is to recognize the fact that pain throughout the joints, combined with psoriasis, does not necessarily spell a diagnosis of psoriatic arthritis. More than likely it does, but it may also mean that there is an underlying condition present that is incidental to the psoriasis. Nevertheless, the treatment is basically the same, whether they are combined or separate conditions.

## Poker Spine

One of the most disabling symptoms occurs when psoriatic arthritis affects the spine—which, in my practice, has been the case with a good number of patients. Of course, there are varying degrees of spinal involvement. The types I have encountered most frequently are those in which there is practically no flexibility of the spine, a condition termed *poker spine.* Manipulating such a spine is like trying to manipulate a steel rod. This is a characteristic feature of conditions such as rheumatoid arthritis of the spine, spondyloarthritis, ankylosing spondylitis, and psoriatic spondylitis.

In long-standing cases, the spine on an X-ray may look like a calcified steel rod, or it may be unremarkable. Either way, the normal range of motion, flexibility, and pliability of the spine is absent. The longitudinal spinal ligaments and soft tissue elements surrounding the vertebrae are so dried up and rigid that movement, even by manipulation, is virtually impossible. Age has little to do with it. I have patients in their twenties whose spines are just as rigid as others with the same problem who are in their sixties.

In this case, the chiropractor or the osteopath must exercise extreme caution by not being too forceful in using downward pressure in an attempt to achieve movement of the spinal motor units. Gentle, steady downward pressure all along the spine, without attempting to adjust anything, is the procedure I follow. The doctor is aiming for improved flexibility, not spinal correction. It is all that can be expected anyway, and the patient will love a practitioner for being gentle in his approach. In time, with the steady use of peanut-oil massages, particularly along the spine, the doctor may feel minor adjustments taking place. With continued conservative manipulation, more flexibility will be established, and in time, a greater range of motion, without pain, will be experienced by the patient. Here is where three stimulating units—the Morfam Master Massager, the Oster Hand Massager, and the electrical stimulation unit (administered by a physician or a physiotherapist)—can be extremely helpful.

In such severe cases, treatment must be expected to continue for a year or more, which is nothing when you consider the alternative. At least something is being done that will help put the condition in check and slowly reverse the disease process. Doing nothing invariably means a continued lifetime of pain, with increasing immobility leading to possible invalidism.

## Some Added Measures

The bottom line in psoriatic arthritis is time, patience, and effort. There is no substitute. It must be remembered that the patient's chemistry is out of balance—even if the myriad serological tests show negative results. Here is a case where the patient's reaction serves as the best barometer in determining the degree of progress.

Since these cases fall within the most severe type of psoriasis known, every form of hydrotherapy (water therapy) should be utilized: steam, whirlpool, colonics, fume baths, swimming (see chapter 9), and yes, one can consider drinking six to eight glasses of pure water a part of internal hydrotherapy.

Controlled modalities such as electrical stimulation as well as roller-type massage units applied along the entire spine can be extremely helpful. *Gentle* stretch exercises are encouraged but must be geared to each individual patient. Sustained stretch positions, such as yoga postures, are very helpful and therapeutic. They also provide a criterion to judge improvement, by increased range of motion.

Finally, as a mental exercise, key words should be visualized and even uttered audibly to oneself. Any terms that signify the goal may be used; for example, *flexibility, rubber, elastic, stretchability, rag doll,* "*loose as a goose,*" and so forth. These power-packed words have more significance than you may think. They represent an attitude, one that is the very opposite of what psoriatic arthritis represents. I advise my patients to "try it—you might like it."

## The Professor's Story

In the years that have passed since the first printing of this book, I have had the experience of treating several psoriatic arthritic patients. The only patients who have succeeded were those who persisted. This is not to say they all were cured, but the treatment most assuredly provided them with a better quality of life: freedom from pain, greater flexibility, and, equally important, relief from anxiety and fear. They make the regimen a way of life, and as many have expressed it, "It's a good way!"

The most severe case that I have cared for in recent years was that of H.W., a college history professor. He was riddled with psoriasis, combined with psoriatic arthritis, to the extent that he was referred to as "the lobster man" at a major New York medical center. General everyday movements were accomplished with severe pain and discomfort, if he was able to do these moves at all. Getting up out of a chair or trying to write on a blackboard for his classes was a traumatic experience. He had been under orthodox management for twenty-eight years, using every method available. He came to me on November 11, 1995, and began the regimen with total commitment from the very start. Every measure was faithfully followed—diet, colonics, oils, spinal adjustments, teas, and so forth, for over a year. By October 1996, he was able to walk briskly over a mile a day, play stickball with his friends again, and flex his arms and hands as if they were made of rubber. Practically every lesion on his body had disappeared. After thirty years, the joy of living was returned to him. The reason for the professor's success is no secret. It took hard work on both our parts. To know what to do is one thing; to carry it out is quite another. He followed through, and nature rewarded him in time, beyond his greatest expectations.

## More on the Leaky Gut Syndrome

In chapter 1 I expounded upon the theory of the leaky gut syndrome as being a basic cause of many degenerative diseases, psoriasis being one of them. This concept, described by Dr. Zoltan P. Rona, of Toronto, Canada, is further strengthened by the works of Leo Galland, MD, in his article titled, "Leaky Gut Syndrome: Breaking the Vicious Cycle," in which he lists not only psoriasis, eczema, and other diseases as having the same cause, but includes arthritis as a clear possibility as well. (For the full text, see www.mdheal.org.)

*Glutamine supplement* has been referred to as an important substrate for the maintenance of the intestinal wall. Feeding glutamine reverses all the abnormalities involved in the breakdown of the intestinal wall, according to Dr. Galland. He maintains that fish oil helps repair the intestinal wall injured by the taking of methotrexate (MTX) and additionally blunts the systemic circulatory response to endotoxins.

## Additional Helpful Suggestions

High on the list of helpful food supplements for the psoriatic arthritic patient is Norwegian cod liver oil with omega-3 polyunsaturates, either in liquid or tablet form. Considerable benefits have been seen in many cases of arthritis that I have encountered. I believe the benefits are derived from the healing effects on the intestinal walls attributed to the omega-3 oils and to the high content of vitamin A. But remember, the best source of omega-3 fish oils is fresh fish itself. The darker and oilier the fish, the better it is.

## Loosen Up!

And last, but by no means least, I advise you to start taking things lightly. I tell sufferers to loosen up mentally as well as physically, to learn to bend with the wind and be less harsh on themselves and on others. The reasoning behind adopting such attitudes is simple when one realizes the eternal truth that a rigid mentality has as its constant companion a rigid body!

# CHAPTER 17

# Cases of Eczema (Atopic Dermatitis)

T he disease that comes closest to simulating psoriasis is eczema. Both diseases produce scales; have reddened, inflamed areas; ooze at times; and can produce an uncontrollable itch that is a living hell for the sufferer. There are even times when a person may have a combination of the two diseases. From the orthodox medical viewpoint, they are considered two separate diseases. From a medical point of view, this is probably best, because the treatments differ. From the Edgar Cayce readings, however, we learn the exact opposite. There most certainly is a correlation between the two diseases, not only in cause, but also in treatment.

During my years of working with psoriasis, a few cases of eczema have come into the office. Admittedly, this hardly constitutes the basis for a valid research report, but when three out of four cases clear up completely by following basically the same regimen I give for psoriasis, something demands our attention.

## The First Case

In December 1979, Mr. R.P. came to me complaining of a severe case of eczema. Having suffered with it for years, he desperately sought a remedy. He had heard of my work with psoriasis through the Association for Research and Enlightenment (ARE) and wondered if I could offer any help. I made it quite clear at our first meeting that I had never encountered a case of eczema and had no experience with it. His desperate plea touched me, however, and I agreed to send for the Cayce file on eczema with the understanding that I would not take R.P.'s case if the therapy did not fall within my scope of practice. With this understanding, we proceeded.

Amazingly, a careful perusal of the eczema discourses revealed such a startling parallel to psoriasis that I was almost convinced they had sent the wrong file. This was not so; it *was* the eczema file. For two weeks I studied and extracted every possible measure that could benefit R.P.

The cause of eczema was listed as the same thinning of the intestinal walls, a supertoxic body accompanied by poor elimination. The adherence to a high-alkaline-producing diet was essential, with proper elimination as the key factor in treatment. Only one external measure, the application of Ray's Ointment or Liquid or Lenoir's Eczema Remedy, was suggested often for eczema and only occasionally for psoriasis. Since they are not prescription items, the patient obtained them on his own. The same slippery elm bark powder, American yellow saffron tea, and mullein tea were the primary herbs suggested for intestinal cleansing. The adjustments of the spine were slightly different. The emphasis was placed on the third and fourth dorsal area, throughout the lumbars, but there was also special reference to the sixth dorsal. The similarity in cause and treatment of eczema and psoriasis was very obvious in the Cayce material.

After I placed R.P. on the same basic regimen as that for psoriasis, he agreed to follow each measure as faithfully as possible. He came to my office for a few visits, but then was unable to return for three months. When he did return, the results were extremely encouraging. For the first time in years, he was enthusiastic, vital, and vibrant, and his skin had improved considerably.

In another month, all discomfort had subsided. Within six months, he was satisfied with the condition of his skin and in all other areas of his life as well. His job endeavors improved slowly but steadily, his skin remained clear, his attitude was extremely positive, and his sense of desperation and anxiety had given way to calmness. He was a relaxed man, in charge of his life again.

On October 29, 1980, I gave a talk on psoriasis in the Dag Hammarskjöld Library Auditorium at the United Nations in New York. As I prepared to go onstage, R.P. came up to inform me that he was in the audience and if I cared to mention his particular case, he would confirm it. An opportunity arose toward the end of my talk, and I presented his case. After I introduced him, he surprised everybody (including me) by exposing his arms and legs, now totally clear of eczema, attributing his success to following the regimen. I had no way of knowing whether this treatment would work in all cases of eczema, but in R.P.'s case, thanks to his self-discipline, it worked indeed.

In the two years following the case of R.P., I had only two other cases of eczema. One was an adorable little girl whose mother followed all instructions conscientiously to another successful outcome. Another was an adult woman who had been suffering from a very severe case of eczema since infancy. I do not consider her response successful, although she improved somewhat after three or four months. She discontinued further treatment in favor of other methods. Perhaps more time would have been needed to cleanse her body internally. One thing, however, stands out in her case history—she had had a lifetime of poor elimination.

## A Case via Telephone

It wasn't until January 1983 that I encountered the next case of eczema. One weekend, A.G., a dear friend of mine from upstate New York, related to me the sad plight of her lifelong friend, Mrs. M.K., who was ninety-two years old. M.K. had been a very active person until 1981, when she developed a harsh case of eczema. The itch throughout her arms was unbearable. Although she had been under the care of two dermatologists during this time, nothing brought her relief, and the condition worsened.

A.G. asked me if there was anything I could do for her friend. I answered it was possible, providing she followed all instructions. A.G. insisted that I call her and discuss the matter, as she was in a desperate state. I called. The voice on the phone was that of a marvelous human being with a deep-rooted, loving philosophy of life that had sustained her positively through the years. Her gratitude for my time was apparent from the beginning of the conversation. She explained that she had been diagnosed by both her dermatologists as having eczema. Even at the age of ninety-two, she would not accept this as her fate or destiny. She knew there was an answer somewhere.

Since the case of R.P. had proven so successful, I was able to convey to M.K. the details of his success, as well as my experience with psoriasis. Dr. Ronald Marks, a leading researcher considered to be an authority on psoriasis, has said, "It is not much good treating someone for psoriasis if what they have is really eczema." This probably holds true from the viewpoint of orthodox treatment, but from the Cayce outlook, I must respond to this fine physician that, in fact, I have found the opposite to be true.

As I dictated the regimen to M.K. over the phone, she took detailed notes and repeatedly said how grateful she was and that she would follow it exactly. When I explained the importance of proper elimination in that there should be no constipation at all, she sighed with relief. She explained, "I told the doctors that I was often constipated, but they would virtually ignore me and made it sound unimportant and unrelated to my problem." I suggested that she take the necessary steps to relieve her constipation problem immediately.

In addition, and of equal importance, I took her off whole milk and placed her on goat's milk. The powdered form is found, or can be ordered, in most health food stores. This determined, enthusiastic woman followed every suggestion to the best of her ability. She sent out for the proper vegetables, juices, herbal teas, and so forth. Within the first month, the condition worsened, as often happens with psoriasis cases as well. Then slowly, a change began to occur. A gradual, steady improvement manifested as the change of diet helped regulate her bowel movements, and elimination was no longer a problem.

A few times, her visiting nurse administered a home enema, which made a decided difference. I advised a regulated diet, especially avoiding foods with a high fat content and excluding nightshades and sweets. Goat's milk became a regular part of her diet. The regimen paid off handsomely, but her strong desire to rid her body of this irritating disease was the overriding factor.

The next time I heard from M.K. was in June 1983, while I was visiting A.G., five months after our initial telephone conversation.

M.K. insisted that I visit her. This I did, and I am happy to relate that a joyful, dignified, elegant lady greeted me at the door. There wasn't a mark or lesion on her. She now enjoyed freedom from that unbearable itch, pain, and stiffness.

She had invited me to visit her, not only to see firsthand the results obtained, but also to thank me personally for putting her on the right track. In appreciation, she gave me one of her prized possessions, a 1936 edition of *Gone with the Wind* signed by the author, Margaret Mitchell, who had been a personal friend of the family.

M.K.'s story is an inspiration to me and all who know her. A woman of ninety-two, instead of giving up, made up her mind to do whatever was required. After receiving instructions over a few phone calls, she was determined to follow through, and she succeeded. For those younger patients with eczema who feel the procedure is too much trouble, I have only pity. The road ahead can be long, tedious, and expensive, and a great deal of pain and effort will be experienced due to an unwillingness to consider this alternative route.

I visited M.K. again in August 1983, on her invitation, to choose all the books I wanted from her library. Before departing her gracious company, I asked the one question I ask of all my successful patients: "Mrs. M.K., what do you believe was the key to getting well?" She thought a moment and, with a twinkle in her eye, looked up at me and said, "Well, Doctor, eloquently speaking, when I stopped being constipated!"

The reader should have a clear appreciation of the similarities in cause and regimen of treatment for psoriasis and eczema. There are, however, a few specific differences in treating eczema as compared to psoriasis. The regimen is basically the same except for the external application of Ray's Ointment for eczema versus Cuticura or hydrophilic ointment for psoriasis. Internally, as an intestinal cleanser, any good natural laxative will do, such as stewed fruits, syrup of figs, Senokot, psyllium husks, and so forth. The only stipulation here is to try to alternate using a laxative with a fruit base with one having a vegetable base. It is best not to use the same type of laxative all the time. Furthermore, I advise cotton fabric not only for bedsheets, but also pajamas and undergarments, especially panty hose. Even bathing suits are best when made of cotton (or mostly cotton), rather than nylon, silk, or spandex. In other words, the eczema patient or psoriatic will do well to avoid any synthetic fabrics clinging to the skin. The more the skin can breathe, the better the results.

## Eczema in Young Children

Always keep in mind that the basic cause of eczema is toxic accumulations in the body, whether the patient is young or old. Poor elimination and improper food selection are the major contributing factors. More than likely, it is a combination of the two. I have found the causes of psoriasis and eczema to be the same. The following measures are suggested, with approval of your pediatrician:

1. Drink plenty of pure water each day (at least 4 to 6 glasses).
2. Adhere to the 70–80 percent/20–30 percent alkaline-acid dietary food chart.
3. Daily take 1 or 2 drops of castor oil added to a glass or bottle of water.
4. Remove 1 teaspoon of liquid from a bottle of Fletcher's Castoria and replace it with 1 teaspoon of olive oil. Shake the bottle well before using. In young children, 1 teaspoon of this mixture is given daily. For those over age five, give 2 teaspoons a day (it is best between meals). As the elimination improves, so will the skin. The child should stop taking the mixture once he or she is clear.
5. Slippery elm tea should be taken in the morning; saffron tea late in the day.
6. External applications help to relieve the severe itching and discomfort. Use castor oil, an olive oil–peanut oil mixture, Lubriderm, or Aveeno anti-itch formula. In some cases, an Aveeno bath helps. Sometimes a soft cloth rinsed out in cool water and applied to the affected area brings considerable relief. For small areas of severe inflammation, wrap an ice cube in a handkerchief and apply directly to the skin to give relief. The application of Johnson's baby powder or cornstarch on the itchy areas, especially at night, has been successful in many cases.
7. The child should have 1 to 3 teaspoons of pure olive oil per day.

8. The child must adhere to the rules of diet, especially:

- No fried foods, for example, potato chips, french fries, doughnuts.
- No nightshades or nightshade products. These are: tomatoes, tobacco, eggplant, white potatoes, peppers (hot spices), and paprika.
- No sweets to any great extent, especially chocolate, candy, cakes, and icing. No corn syrup or products made with corn syrup. (Read labels.)
- Avoid milk and milk products as much as possible; try skim milk, soy milk, or goat's milk instead of whole milk.
- Avoid any food item that causes an allergic reaction.

Remember, the purpose of the external application is to merely calm the skin down and make the patient more comfortable during the healing process, which is taking place on the inside.

## "Little Boy on Fire!"

In March 1994, Mr. and Mrs. T.P. called, desperately seeking an answer for two-year-old M.P.'s condition. He had been described, by at least four dermatologists, as being "the worst case of infantile eczema they had ever seen." It began when he was two months of age. When I saw the boy for the first time, on March 25, 1994, the reason for the parents' anxiety was obvious. Little M.P.'s head and arms looked as though he had suffered third-degree burns. His screams, restlessness, and pain made me wonder if anything at all could be done, since he failed to respond to the various dermatologists' treatment. But we had to try. With total commitment to the regimen for young children, M.P.'s parents began the procedure. Within days, encouraging changes were seen. The next week showed continued improvement: no scales or scabs. After nine months, the final big breakthrough occurred, and M.P. steadily healed. I saw him a total of two times. It was his parents' devotion that pulled him through.

M.P.'s case is presented in the photographs on page 245, as an example of what is possible in such cases when knowledge of the procedure is followed through with consistency and persistence. It should inspire every parent, guardian, and even a child old enough to understand, as to the effectiveness of this regimen.

A letter from M.P.'s mother reads:

You've helped M.P. so much when he suffered so severely with eczema. Look at him today—6 years old and going into the first grade. Looking forward to your newest edition.

D.P.

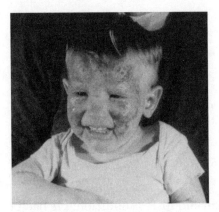

M.P., age 2, at the start of the regimen.

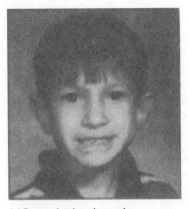

M.P., age 6, a handsome boy.

Throughout the years that followed, I used these principles on several small children, with similar results. Some take longer than others to heal, and some have flare-ups along the way, but with such an approach, results are very promising. I pass this information on to my readers, not because it provides a guarantee of favorable results in every case, but because the event was true and may very well prove to be a godsend when all else fails for some children suffering with eczema.

## The Correlation between Psoriasis and Eczema

Other differences are minor, but for the reader's interest, I have listed below a comparative view of both conditions, followed by some appropriate dietary measures.

**PSORIASIS**

(Gk., *psora:* to have the itch)

1. Basically a toxemia
2. Cause: poor elimination, thinning of intestinal walls
3. Blood: excess acidity
4. Cathartics (laxatives):
   - Innerclean
   - Senokot
   - Olive oil
   - Psyllium husks
   - Milk of magnesia
   - Fletcher's Castoria
   - Castor oil
5. External applications:
   - Creamy Vaseline
   - Cuticura ointment
   - Castor oil
   - Hydrophilic ointment
   - Olive oil/peanut oil

**ECZEMA**

(Gk., *ekzema:* to boil, ferment)

1. Basically a toxemia
2. Cause: poor elimination, thinning of intestinal walls
3. Blood: excess acidity
4. Cathartics (laxatives):
   - Innerclean
   - Senokot
   - Olive oil
   - Psyllium husks
   - Milk of magnesia
   - Fletcher's Castoria
   - Castor oil
5. External applications:
   - Ray's Ointment
   - Lenoir's Eczema Remedy
   - Olive oil–peanut oil
   - Noxzema
   - Johnson's baby powder

6. Spinal adjustments (in order of importance):

   - Sixth, seventh, and ninth dorsal
   - Third cervical
   - Throughout the lumbars, especially especially the fourth

7. Sources of irritation:

   - Duodenum
   - Jejunum
   - Upper intestinal tract

8. Recommended:

   - High colonic irrigations (not for children under fourteen), followed by Glyco-Thymoline (diluted) as a final rinse
   - Home enemas

9. Diet should be highly alkaline.

10. Fish, fowl, and lamb (never fried) are permitted.

11. No alcohol (red wine as a food is okay).

12. Skim or low-fat milk and/or buttermilk are permitted.

13. Drink six to eight glasses of pure water daily.

14. Sunshine usually helps, but avoid sunburn.

15. Undergarments and bed linens should be made of cotton or have a high cotton content.

16. If on hands, wear protective gloves when washing dishes or working with solvents.

6. Spinal adjustments (in order of importance):

   - Third, fourth, sixth, and ninth dorsal
   - Third cervical
   - Throughout the lumbars, especially especially the fourth

7. Sources of irritation:

   - Stomach
   - Duodenum/jejunum
   - Upper intestinal tract

8. Recommended:

   - High colonic irrigations (not for children under fourteen), followed by Glyco-Thymoline (diluted) as a final rinse
   - Home enemas

9. Diet should be highly alkaline.

10. Fowl and lamb, occasionally fish (never fried), well masticated, are permitted.

11. No alcohol (red wine, but no more than 4 ounces daily, is okay).

12. Goat's milk or soy milk is preferred.

13. Drink six to eight glasses of pure water daily.

14. Sunshine usually helps, but avoid sunburn.

15. Undergarments and bed linens should be made of cotton or have a high cotton content.

16. If on hands, wear protective gloves when washing dishes or working with solvents.

*Note:* Products such as Innerclean, Ray's Ointment, an olive oil–peanut oil mixture, and Glyco-Thymoline can be obtained through the Cayce suppliers listed in appendix D.

### Treatment Factors in Common: Psoriasis and Eczema

1. Eat plenty of green leafy vegetables, especially watercress, celery, and lettuce.

2. American yellow saffron tea and mullein tea are called for in both. Drink plenty of water and no carbonated beverages.

3. The perspiratory glands become more active in both cases when there is a lack of coordination in the eliminating system; therefore, synthetic undergarments, especially those that cling to the skin, are to be avoided. Preferred are undergarments and bed linens made entirely from cotton or with a high percentage of cotton.

4. Maintain a cheerful disposition. Smile, for to worry or become cross and antagonistic creates poisons, just as much as the wrong foods do.

5. Slippery elm bark powder taken in water five days of the week is a good general rule for both.

6. Independent research has shown that two to four tablespoons of granular lecithin each day is extremely helpful in treating both psoriasis and eczema.

7. Do not eat any nightshades in either case, especially tomatoes, and no hot spices, vinegar, shellfish, and peanuts or any tree nut that a person may be allergic to. Animal fats should be cut down considerably. Fish, fowl, and lamb are permitted, but never fried. Remember, the darker and oilier the fish, the better. Do not eat french fries or any other fried foods. The dietary measures for eczema, in general, are the same as those suggested for psoriasis. It cannot be overemphasized that diet and internal cleansing are the key factors in alleviating eczema as well as psoriasis. In the case of eczema, however, keep fruits and fruit juices to an absolute minimum.

Some dermatologists have suggested that oolong tea can be very helpful in cases of eczema. A study reported in the January 2001 issue of *Archives of Dermatology* of more than one hundred patients with atopic dermatitis demonstrated that drinking a liter of oolong tea daily could dramatically decrease inflammation and itching.

I have no answer as to why one person gets eczema while another gets psoriasis, if the cause is the same. That can be determined only by detailed scientific investigation, if at all. Perhaps they are different forms of the same disease, but someone in authority placed separate labels on them, and, as a result, they are viewed as different diseases. Such a precept can put you off the track from the start.

One factor of considerable importance, which characterizes the study of the Cayce material, is that several different diseases are basically treated the same way, with satisfactory results reported in many cases. This seems to be especially true in the classification of degenerative diseases such as psoriasis, arthritis, scleroderma, and other systemic problems. It is as though the body is telling us, "Set me right, feed me correctly, expect me to get well, and I'll heal myself."

It has been my experience to treat a number of these seemingly different health problems. The basic principles of the psoriasis regimen were followed, and a successful outcome was often the result.

# CHAPTER 18

# What about the Failures?

To imply that I have always succeeded with a patient would be not only an exaggeration, but an inexcusable lie. Certainly there have been failures. Some are easily explained; others are not. The reasons remain elusive if the focus is placed only on the regimen and not on the patient as well. The question is, what caused the failure? Did the therapy fail, or did the patient (and the doctor) fail the therapy? Until this question is answered honestly, one cannot judge if the regimen really does or does not work on a specific individual. This I can say unequivocally: if the patient is sincere, follows through faithfully, allows adequate time for the procedure to work, and is willing to change his lifestyle (particularly his eating habits), then the chances of success are greatly enhanced.

Just by the law of averages, however, there is a certain percentage of people who will not respond to this or any other therapy, even if they follow it to the letter. It's anybody's guess why this occurs. Allowing for this unexplained percentage of failure, the one common cause ascribed to most failures is the patient stopped following the regimen.

At times the reason was clear—results were not fast enough. With others, desire for alcoholic drinks, sweets, or rich foods overpowered the desire to clear the skin. And there were some whose cases were simply not severe enough to motivate them to muster up the necessary discipline, especially regarding diet. Even with these unsuccessful cases, most of them showed some degree of improvement. *Persistence* is the key word in the treatment of psoriasis, as it is in any successful endeavor.

## "Advice" from the Uninformed

Another problem the patient, as well as the physician, must guard against is discouraging thoughts and comments from well-meaning but uninformed relatives and friends. This is why I strongly encourage new patients to bring a close relative or a friend to the initial consultation. There is nothing like evidence, a track record of successful cases, and knowledge of the entire procedure to convert a concerned friend into a helping hand to the patient. There have been countless times when the patient came alone for the initial interview and left the office encouraged and filled with enthusiasm, only to be discouraged by people who took neither the time nor the interest to investigate the process themselves. The psoriatic doesn't need this type of influence. At times, it might be better for the patient not to say anything, proceed with the regimen, and later, if successful, reveal the source of his or her accomplishment.

Naturally, no one wishes to be diseased any longer than necessary, especially with something as miserable as psoriasis. The disease did not develop overnight. Therefore, it follows that it cannot be eliminated overnight. Here is where encouragement comes in.

Part of the physician's responsibility, as well as that of relatives and friends, is to constantly provide the patient with that encouragement to strengthen his or her resolve to get well. Arranging personal introductions between successful patients and new ones is one of the most valuable steps the doctor can take to further promote confidence and assurance. (Of course, permission is first obtained from all parties.)

It takes time to get sick, especially with a systemic-type disease. Although this idea is logical, it is sometimes hard for a patient to grasp that it will also take time to get well. If the condition is not irreversible, and the proper measures are employed, it is amazing how quickly the body will bring itself into equilibrium. This point is stressed with new patients, as much as are diet and other elements of the regimen.

# A Most Irritating Problem

There is nothing more frustrating and mind-boggling than seeing some people struggle for the slightest improvement while others clear up in practically no time at all. Patience is a virtue, and no researcher should be without it, but in all honesty, this is one of the most irritating problems I have had to face in caring for a psoriasis patient.

There have been countless times when I was ready to throw in the towel and go on to newer and more promising things, when all at once a severe case would quickly clear up. This would encourage me until my newly found energy and enthusiasm was thwarted by new failures. I often asked myself why this happened. If this process is real and the principles are followed faithfully, shouldn't the right results *always* be attained?

I believe the answer lies, for one reason or another, within the patients themselves. The successful cases are really the forerunners for further research. I have always maintained that if you want to be successful, you should do what successful people do. Although I prefer to concentrate on those who succeed, there is a certain amount of comfort in observing the failures, for therein you may find a clue as to which direction to avoid.

Thomas A. Edison, the American inventor of many vitally useful products, advocated the value of failure—but only as a catalyst to persist until the answer was found. He must have done something right, for in his eighty-four years (1847–1931), Edison took out 1,093 patents, the most ever granted to any one person. As the practical-minded giver of light, Edison became the American Prometheus, the prophet of technological progress. When asked what he would request from Aladdin's genie if he had the chance, he answered without hesitation, "My health!"

Something can indeed be said for failure, provided it acts as a stimulus to continue to forge ahead with determination to find an answer. The question in my mind is no longer whether the procedures work if they are followed. The question now is, why does it work on some but not on others? I postulate that if it works on one, it has the potential to work on all. With this in mind, the ability of the practitioner to recognize each and every patient as an individual entity is paramount in that person's case management. One must follow the principles practiced by the patients who had a successful outcome. The cardinal rule is to tailor these principles to meet the needs of each patient.

## Reasons for Failure

There are causes for failures as well as for successes. To repeat the question, if many people completely succeed with this regimen, why do others fail? The most common reasons for failure, according to my observations, are the following:

- Inability or lack of determination on the part of the patient to follow through for a long enough period.
- Discouragement from relatives, friends, and physicians unacquainted with this manner of therapy.
- Lack of support and cooperation by the patient's spouse or guardian in preparing the proper foods as outlined.
- X—the unknown. There are always failures that defy explanation. We have had our share, but fortunately, their number represents a small minority.

## Do What Successful People Do

As mentioned earlier, I subscribe to the philosophy that if you want to be successful, study the lives of successful people. Those patients who have succeeded followed every measure of the regimen to the best of their abilities and placed getting well uppermost in their minds. For instance, it never mattered to them what friends might say at a cocktail party if they drank ice water or seltzer with lime on the rocks instead of a highball. They took the time to study a menu while dining out and chose only permitted foods. They prepared their herbal teas each day, took their Epsom salts baths, and had spinal adjustments, as recommended. They were guided by the philosophy "Keep on keeping on!" until the desired results were achieved.

## Sweets and Alcohol

Two things seem to be the most difficult for patients to give up or at least greatly curtail—sweets and alcohol. Excessive smoking is not far behind. Candy is the leading culprit among sweets. Hard alcohol (gin, whiskey, vodka) or excessive quantities of beer is the problem with drinkers. In truth, many patients I have encountered who have one or both of these addictions have a very difficult time abstaining from them. Fortunately, these cases are a minority. Most patients do, in fact, place the clearing of their skin first. Those with the addictions, unless they learn to control their desires, face a lifetime of doctors, expense, and misery.

## They Won't Believe It

One irritating attitude, fortunately rare, is that of patients who after suffering for years with massive lesions covering their bodies, refuse to admit or believe that it was this regimen that cleared them. One patient's girlfriend once called me secretly to tell me, "Doctor, I know it was the diet that completely cleared his skin, but he refuses to believe it and went back to his old way of eating, and he is covered again."

It's puzzling to me why a patient would suddenly go off the diet, knowing it could harm him or at least retard the cleansing process. While I was searching for a logical answer, a successful psoriasis case came forth that made sense to me and to several patients when I brought it to their attention.

It is because, as expressed by one particular patient, "You feel like you are in jail. You can't do this, you can't do that; you can't eat this, you can't eat that." Frustration sets in, but with one big difference—you can always open the door and walk out. A true prisoner does not have that option. When this patient opened the door and walked out, her psoriasis came back. It was then that she realized she did indeed have control over the situation. Once she overcame her "childish" attitude, as she put it, and followed the rules, she was free once again. Her skin cleared and remains as clear as she wants it to be.

Some patients attribute the results to exposure to the sun or ultraviolet treatments but not to the discipline of the dietary requirements and cleansing methods described here. They are stymied, however, when I have them meet patients who completely cleared up without having exposed themselves to the sun or ultraviolet therapy of any kind.

I believe most of these patients feel secure by holding a negative view because that is their habitual way of thinking, and they do not like changing their lifestyle or giving up, even for a short time, their favorite food and drink. Then again, maybe they have been through so much from an orthodox-treatment point of view that they refuse to believe the answer could be so simple.

It is not unusual for some patients with a severe degree of psoriasis to quit this regimen in midstream even when results are beginning to become apparent. Another frustrating experience for the doctor is when positive changes in the skin are seen and the patient admits to it and progress is confirmed by the spouse, but then the patient goes back to his or her old lifestyle, knowing full well the lesions will return—and they do! It seems the patient simply wanted to test this procedure to see if it really worked. Such people appear to adopt the attitude, "Okay, it works—so eventually I'll get around to it. In the meantime, I'll eat and drink what I want." Fortunately, when such rare incidents occur the reason is obvious: lack of discipline concerning diet. Such patients would like to rid themselves of psoriasis, but they consider the price too high. It is incredible what they will suffer in terms of inconvenience, embarrassment, or disfigurement to satisfy their food cravings. Such patients are headed for difficult times if they refuse to change their heart and mind.

I have heard some patients who claim, "My psoriasis just went away and never came back." I have no reason to disbelieve that. But such incidents are extremely rare. To those who wait for it to just go away, I say, "Don't count on it!" Take the action steps to conquer the disease and stop being "childish" about it. Then, and only then, will they have control, if not a complete cure, of the disease.

## "Intellectualizing"—a Pitfall?

Mr. H.M. had a severe case of psoriasis on his face (which is rather rare), his back, his chest, and particularly his legs. He came to my office seeking any method to stop this progression, which had started only six months earlier. He was a kind, likable, cheerful, hardworking individual. Frankly, I wasn't convinced within myself that he would be successful because he wasn't "intellectual" enough about it. He didn't question the procedure. With the invaluable aid of his wife, he simply followed the instructions to the letter. Within three months, he was completely clear throughout his face, chest, back, and most of his arms, with some remaining lesions disappearing on his legs. Three months later, he was 100 percent clear. When I asked him, as I do all my successful cases, what he thought was the cause of his psoriasis, he quickly answered, "Junk food—you said stay away from it, so I did!"

The "intellectuals" who question everything rather than practice the procedure called for are still battling their skin problem. Mind you, I am not against the person who seeks answers to questions. But I am annoyed by the person who seeks answers that fit his preconceived notions, and, when the answers don't fit, dismisses them.

William Kearny Carr said it best in *The Concurrence:*

> However much intellect is to be commended, it has its disadvantage, since it increases our doubts, and, therefore, becomes the greatest hindrance to our success. All progress is from below, upward; hence we should expect to hear wisdom from the humble and unintelligent. They have not their intellect trained so as to doubt, and hence they often see intuitively and instantly what so often comes laboriously, if at all, to the better disciplined intellect.

Therefore, if the patients will get out of their own way and sincerely seek answers, answers are provided. Again I must emphasize that the success of this or any other worthwhile accomplishment must be founded on the building blocks of *patience and persistence.* Without these two mental ingredients, the structure upon which this principle of healing is based will crumble. This approach is the very opposite of the "quick fix" that so many psoriasis sufferers are looking for. Until they view psoriasis as a systemic problem that must be managed systemically, successful results are difficult, if not impossible, to attain. Once they see this overall picture of the problem, their approach to the disease takes on a new dimension and, if practiced faithfully, usually brings the desired result.

# CHAPTER 19

# The Question of Recurrence

The question of whether psoriasis will return after it clears is, and should be, of primary concern to the patient. Obviously, one would not look enthusiastically upon a mode of therapy that offered only fleeting results—yet, this is often the case in orthodox management.

There are two reasons psoriasis may return after it has been cleared: (1) The root cause of the disease remains, or (2) the patient returns to his or her old way of life too soon. In my observation, the latter is the major reason for the recurrence.

If the psoriasis clears by following this regimen in the first place, we can safely assume we have attacked the primary cause successfully. Therefore, if it returns, the only logical conclusion is that the patient reactivated the primary cause of the disease. What is the solution? It is simple—return to the basic regimen.

Although I mentioned this before, it deserves repetition: once patients clear their skin of psoriasis by following this regimen, they never fear the disease again. That is not to say they will never break out again. They most certainly can and usually do if they grossly abuse their diet. The reason they no longer fear it is that, to a large extent, they now know how to control it on their own. I have often observed patients on their first visit, gripped by apprehension, visualizing themselves getting progressively worse, subject all their lives to periodic hospitalization and ultimately possible invalidism. The whole scene changes, however, when they get well, with not a mark on their bodies, and confidently revert to some of their favorite eating habits with the attitude, "Well, if it pops out again, I'll just go on the diet." There is nothing wrong with that—as long as they never let it get out of hand again. This is how effective it has been for some patients. With others, there seems to be no return at all, regardless of how much they stray from the diet, but this is not usually the case.

I can only surmise with these apparently successful cases that they stayed on the regimen long enough to allow proper and effective healing of the thin intestinal walls. There is no question that they can now live with it, or shall I say without it—and happily at that!

# Updates

In the September 1977 *ARE Journal,* my work in psoriasis appeared for the first time in a feature article titled "Psoriasis—Hope for the Afflicted." In this account, I reported on cases that had cleared and stayed clear for a three- to four-month period. An adequate amount of time had not yet elapsed before publication to observe whether there were to be any truly promising results as far as recurrence was concerned.

That was fourteen years before the first edition of this book. Surely, I would say, that is a reasonable amount of time to observe the validity of the treatment. The following are updates of these patients regarding their present state of health. Photographs of their conditions appeared in chapter 2.

These are but a few of my early cases with a follow-up study several years after they were cleared. Their stories are heartwarming to say the least, offering true hope for those afflicted, especially in the cases of children.

## The Case of William (Bill) Culmone

Mr. Culmone, you may remember, was the first patient ever to follow the Cayce regimen under my care. After battling psoriasis for fifteen years, he followed the prescribed course as my first experiment and completely cleared in three months (from July 25, 1975, to October 16, 1975).

In a communication to me five months after we started treatments, Mrs. Culmone wrote the following:

> Bill's psoriasis has cleared completely as a result of following the five points mentioned, in conjunction with the office treatments (spinal adjustments). Bill was away ten days and did not take any medication with him. He followed his diet somewhat but did not have the sun, oil, colonic or herb treatments. We wanted to see if the psoriasis would return. To date it has not returned. It is now just over five months since his first treatment. No signs of recurrence have been indicated. I, Minnie Culmone, wife of Bill, attest that we followed the treatments for psoriasis and the above statement is true.

After a period of one and one-half years, Mr. Culmone was still clear. He remained completely clear of psoriasis until his death several years later.

## The Case of Young E.L.

E.L. also cleared completely in a period of three to four months and has virtually remained clear after nine years. She is aware of eating the proper foods but, again, strays now and then, without any significant recurrence.

## The Case of B.K.

This was truly one of the most severe cases I have ever encountered. Practically every area of her body was severely afflicted. After suffering for two years, she cleared up in four months. Her thighs, elbows, scalp, and especially her heels and the soles of her feet seemed to clear simultaneously. After ten years, she reported to me that she has never been troubled with the disease again. What slight flare-ups she might have at times are quickly resolved by going on the cleansing diet again. She has always been in control of her condition since she first cleared in 1977.

# Teenagers, Take Heart!

One does not have to be a child psychologist to know that it is no fun being a young person with psoriasis. Their greatest fear is that they will have to spend the rest of their lives going from one doctor to another, periodically being hospitalized in severe cases, and never able to express their true personalities because of the inhibitions placed on them by the self-consciousness that accompanies psoriasis. Such a reaction is perfectly normal, for no one with a healthy mind wants to hide from life. Yet they do hide to avoid embarrassment and thoughtless remarks from some of their peers.

A particular frustration is not being able to partake of junk food with their friends. They may feel like an outcast, which, in turn, leads to even greater disappointment and undoubtedly produces internal toxins of their own accord. A vicious cycle is established: you're damned if you do and damned if you don't.

With some teenagers, however, depending on their attitude, there is no problem. True, they would like to enjoy the same foods and drinks as their friends, but they also understand and recognize the reason for their particular problem, so they stay away from such foods and avoid making it an issue. The strangest thing of all, however, is that after the first time or two in which they select only the foods that are permitted, their friends don't care. If they are harassed at first, an answer which has proven effective is, "I'd like to have that, but at the moment, I'm on a special physical fitness diet." If the patient makes light of it, so will his or her friends. This produces a twofold benefit: they eat the proper foods and also realize that they are just as well liked by their friends for showing their individuality.

Do they still have to look upon the rest of their lives filled with so many restrictions, particularly diet? Not necessarily. At the present time, I am coming closer to believing that, at least in some cases, the dietary restrictions can be lifted, almost permanently, if the patient stays on the regimen for at least six months after he clears. This fact has been mentioned in other chapters throughout this book, but the following account, written by the mother of a teenager, B.M., who suffered a severe case of guttate psoriasis all over her body, should make teenagers take heart.

My daughter B. started treatment with Dr. Pagano on January 7, 1983, after months of going to allergists and dermatologists. She was thirteen at the time and had psoriasis all over her body, on her head, and on her face. The other doctors told me she would have to learn to live with it, and gave me creams to put on her skin, which did not help. It is very hard for a thirteen-year-old to be told to live with such a disfigurement.

After six months of treatment with Dr. Pagano, she cleared up, but then went off her diet and broke out again. She then resumed treatment and stayed on her diet. It has been two years since she cleared up, with no recurrence. She also can eat anything she wants. Not a day goes by that I do not feel eternally grateful.

## Having It Your Own Way

All psoriatics must keep in mind that they still may have a *tendency* toward the disease, even if every lesion on their body disappears through following this regimen. This should not be upsetting, and it usually isn't, for as stated earlier, the patients now have an understanding as to why it occurs and know what they must do to correct it. They can live free of the disease and live normal lives, provided they are willing to admit that their system reacts differently from others' systems, particularly where certain foods are concerned. This is not unlike the experience of a diabetic or an alcoholic; the difference being that psoriasis is far more controllable than diabetes or alcoholism. They must learn to work with that fact, rather than fight it, for if they don't, they will be fighting a losing battle. To insist on an attitude of "I want what I want when I want it" is to seal their destiny to a lifetime of pain, disfigurement, mental anguish, and incredible expense. Instead, they should adopt the healthful attitude of "I will do all that is required of me" and be thankful there is a way out of their dilemma. If they do, chances are in their favor that they will never again be concerned with the question of recurrence.

# CHAPTER 20

# Achieving the Goal: A Mini-Review

Before embarking on a regimen for the alleviation of any disease, I believe it is essential for the patient to understand not only the nature of the condition, but also the reasoning behind the course of therapy. By way of review, I advise my patients to always keep the following principles in mind:

1. Recognize psoriasis for what it is: the external manifestation of accumulated internal toxins.

2. The way to conquer the disease is to remove the toxins that have accumulated and to prevent further contaminants from entering the system.

3. Toxins are removed and pollution is averted primarily by internal cleansing and proper dietary selection of food and drink.

Other measures that help heal the intestinal walls, such as herbal teas, spinal adjustments, oils, colonics, the right mental attitude, and so forth, aid this process and will help to achieve the goal of attaining clear skin in the shortest possible time. The following is the basic procedure that I use for most of my patients, altering as needed.

## The Apple Diet (the Initial Cleansing)

Each day, for a period of three days, patients eat nothing but Red or Golden Delicious apples (approximately six to eight) and drink six to eight glasses of pure water. In addition, they take one to two ounces of pure olive oil each night, followed by an enema.

On the third day, a colonic irrigation should be administered, if possible. Enemas may be given if colonics are unavailable. This is the most effective way to begin the internal cleansing process. For details, refer to chapter 5.

After having the colonic, patients have a pint of plain yogurt. A few hours later, they eat a large green leafy salad. Dressing may be used, but wine and grain vinegar are avoided. The dressing most preferred is olive oil combined with fresh lemon juice.

*Note:* The apple diet is not for everyone. Check with your physician first.

## The Diet

The dietary measures are continued as detailed in chapter 6. Remember, *diet* and *proper eliminations* are the most important aspects of the regimen. Drinking six to eight glasses of pure water daily is essential. (*Note:* The easiest way to practice the principles of the regimen is to follow the recipes specifically designed for psoriatics and presented in my cookbook, *Dr. John's Healing Psoriasis Cookbook . . . Plus!* available online at www.psoriasis-healing.com.)

## Epsom Salts Baths and Oils

Hot Epsom salts baths can be taken two or three times a week. However, this is not advised if you suffer from any kind of heart or circulatory condition or have skin with open sores that are cracked or sensitive.

An Epsom salts bath is to be followed by an olive oil–peanut oil massage, with the oils left on for at least one-half to one hour. The best results are achieved by leaving the oils on overnight. Wearing old or inexpensive cotton garments over the oils has been found to be both comfortable and practical.

For thick, circumscribed lesions, castor oil rubbed well into these areas, followed by an application of Cuticura or hydrophilic ointment, has, in most cases, proven to be very effective. These products should be used daily until results are obtained. When improvement occurs, the patient cuts back to applying these substances every other day. They discontinue use when the skin is cleared up. For more information, review chapter 9.

## Herbal Teas

Slippery elm bark powder and American yellow saffron tea are the primary herbal teas recommended. The alternatives are chamomile, mullein, and watermelon seed teas, which may be substituted periodically for the saffron tea.

Slippery elm bark powder is to be taken first thing in the morning. For severe cases, I have my patients drink it each morning for ten days, then every other morning for the next two weeks. Sometimes I have them refrain from taking it at all for the next full week. This cycle is repeated until clearing takes place. In mild cases, it is taken every other day for three weeks and not on the fourth week. Again, the patient is to repeat this cycle until results are obtained. (*Note:* Slippery elm is not advised for pregnant women or those contemplating pregnancy.)

American yellow saffron tea is to be taken in the afternoon and into the evening. A cup or two of freshly prepared saffron tea during this period is advised for mild cases. For severe cases, in addition to the tea, a teaspoon of saffron tea is mixed into a gallon of pure water, producing saffron water. It is used as the patient's drinking water whenever desired. As the lesions clear, it is no longer necessary to drink saffron water. However, the patient should still have a cup or two of saffron tea in the evening. (*Note:* American yellow saffron tea is not advised for pregnant women or those contemplating pregnancy.)

If, for any reason, a patient cannot drink the slippery elm tea early in the morning, he or she may drink it at bedtime and have the saffron tea in the morning and throughout the day. Chapter 7 details the preparation of these teas as I advise my patients.

## Spinal Adjustments

Spinal adjustments are usually administered after the first colonic, and this process is to be continued once a week for twelve weeks. The treatments are centered on the sixth and seventh dorsal, the third cervical, the ninth dorsal, and the fourth lumbar vertebrae. They are to be adjusted only by a licensed chiropractor or osteopath. Stubborn cases will require a continuation of treatments until results are obtained. For full details, refer to chapter 8.

# The Thought Process

The correct psychology for getting well must always be the underlying common denominator for healing, especially when the patient is largely in control of his or her own regimen. Correct thinking and guarding one's thoughts from negative outside influences play a vital role in recovery. Make no mistake about it: mental toxins in the form of anxiety, fear, resentment, and so forth can turn the body acidic just as surely as acid-forming foods do—even more so. Chapters 10 and 11 reinforce this concept.

## Remembering the Purpose behind Each of the Six Basic Suggestions

| SUGGESTION | PURPOSE |
| --- | --- |
| 1. *Internal cleansing:* Enemas; high colonics; fume, steam, and Epsom salts baths; cathartics (laxatives); plenty of fresh water. | To remove accumulated toxins (poisons) by improved bowel evacuation, adequate urinary drainage, and through the pores of the skin itself. |
| 2. *The proper diet:* High alkaline (80 percent) to low acid (20 percent); high fiber, fresh fruit and vegetables in particular. | Tends to keep the body chemistry more alkaline than acid. Helps improve eliminations as well as body building. |
| 3. *Herbal teas:* Primarily slippery elm bark powder and American yellow saffron tea (substitutes for saffron tea: chamomile, mullein, and watermelon seed tea). | Slippery elm aids in the healing and rebuilding of the thin intestinal walls and helps prevent absorption of toxins. Saffron helps in the repair of intestinal walls, acts as an intestinal antiseptic, flushes out the liver and the kidneys, and removes toxins through the perspiratory (sweat) glands if taken prior to a steam bath. |

*(Continued)*

### Remembering the Purpose behind Each of the Six
### Basic Suggestions *(continued)*

| SUGGESTION | PURPOSE |
| --- | --- |
| 4. *Spinal adjustments:* Centered on (in order of importance) sixth and seventh dorsal, third cervical, nineth dorsal, and fourth lumbar vertebrae. | Ensures proper nerve impulses and circulation to the walls of the upper intestinal tract, as well as the glandular centers. |
| 5. *External applications:* Oils, ointments, baths, steam, massage. | Help soothe the external lesions, keeping them soft and pliable. Help reduce scaling, relieve itching, and heal the surface cells. |
| 6. *Right thinking* | Helps keep the mind focused on the healing process rather than on the disease. |

Each patient is advised to "see" in his mind's eye the purpose for each suggestion actually taking place as it is carried out. This practice, called visualization, aids the healing process.

Patience and persistence are the keys to all the aforementioned procedures. Without these factors, you cannot even hope to achieve a satisfactory result, especially one that is lasting. It is important to keep in mind just how long you have struggled and lived with this disease and how much psoriasis has dominated your life. The patients who have been successful in managing their condition by following the prescribed regimen feel that the time they spent and the sacrifices they have made to rid themselves of this disease are a tiny price to pay to have this burden lifted from their shoulders.

# CHAPTER 21

# Where Do We Go from Here?

The photographic results depicted in this book have more significance than meets the eye. Of course, first and foremost, they prove that the theory works for many people. Just as profound is the fact that these results were obtained under the worst conditions. By that I mean there was no direct daily control. The patients were told what to do and were expected to go home and do it. Except for the spinal adjustments once a week, which could take place only in the office, the patients were largely on their own.

## Needed: The Ideal Psoriasis Center

On each visit, progress was noted, concepts were reinforced, and, whenever possible, personal meetings with other successful patients were arranged. I mark this fact as significant in that if results such as those depicted herein were possible without complete control, how much more successful would they be under hospital or clinical auspices? All the measures would be administered with the proper equipment, ingredients, attitude, and environment. Ideally, such a center should be located near the sea, where there is plenty of fresh air and sunshine, and be as pollution-free as possible.

Patients would come to such a center to learn as well as to have the therapies administered over a two- to four-week period. After the patient's initial stay, he would have the knowledge of how to handle his problem and would return home to continue to carry out the procedures.

A two- to four-week stay might show a significant change in the skin, but not necessarily. Chances are, the change would not be as dramatic as PUVA or the Goeckerman treatment, which have been shown to apparently clear the skin almost completely in that period of time—in some cases, with results remaining for many months. In just as many cases, however, the condition returned shortly afterward and in full force, usually worse than before. Desperation is the understandable aftereffect, not to mention the fact that with such therapy, the patient is always dependent on hospital control.

I believe a psoriasis center would be much in demand and highly valuable to the psoriatic. *Patience* and *persistence* in *all* matters may one day make such a center a reality.

## The Future—a Choice

Let's say the patients have followed the regimen and are successful. The lesions have completely disappeared. Their skin is beautiful. They feel confident and proud of themselves. What now? Will psoriasis return? Are they really cured of the malady, or will it hang over their heads forever?

The answer to these questions depends a great deal on how one interprets the word *cure.* Blakiston's *New Gould Medical Dictionary* defines *cure* as "to heal or make well." It is the successful treatment of an illness or a wound.

To be cured of a disease does not mean it could never return, particularly if the patient resumes the lifestyle or conditions that brought it about in the first place. It means the malady has been corrected—that, obviously, the course of therapy employed was effective in bringing about healing.

In cases of psoriasis, the patient does have a choice. This is not necessarily true for all diseases. He or she may choose to ignore the basic rules of proper hygiene and sound reasoning pertaining to his former illness and bring about a resurgence of the problem, or he or she could react with gratitude, respect his or her body, appreciate it, and learn to prevent further episodes of ill health for the remainder of his or her life. This, to me, is the person who is "cured." The healing was physically, mentally, and spiritually complete.

Most of the cases that I have successfully treated later fall into one or a combination of the following categories:

*Group I*. They will be eternally grateful and remain on the regimen practically as a way of life and, more than likely, will always remain clear.

*Group II*. They will remain faithful to the basic regimen "for the most part," but will periodically eat whatever they enjoy.

This attitude prevails with the majority of patients, and I am not necessarily against it. Let's face it—we want to enjoy our lives; food and drink is part of that enjoyment. With some, however, living to eat far overshadows eating to live. Satisfying one's desire for certain foods may prevent frustration from setting in, which, in itself, is a leading cause of toxic buildup with emotional origins. With this group, however, panic no longer exists. They know what works to rid themselves of lesions the minute they begin to appear.

*Group III*. They realize their condition can be completely alleviated, so they go back to their old ways of eating and drinking. In time, the lesions will return, usually worse than before. As with Group II, they won't panic. Having been successful once, they feel they can take over and be in control whenever they decide to get around to it. The sad thing about this group is they never do. These patients get no sympathy from me. They seem to forget that there is a law of irreversibility. One day, the organs of the emunctory system will, because of overtaxation, break down to the point of no return.

This group should hear as often as I do the pleas of those who live with them and suffer the silent burden of "cleanup" wherever the psoriatic goes. How often I have heard, "Doctor, every day, all day, to keep my home presentable, I have to follow my husband around with a vacuum cleaner. In the morning, I scoop up scales in our bed as I would scoop up snow or sand on the beach. It is driving me crazy."

True, the psoriasis patient has a problem, but so do those who live with him or her. To some devoted and sincere people, complaining about their loved one's condition seems selfish, so they refrain from voicing their true feelings. Complaining in this regard, however, is nothing compared to the selfishness of the patient who chooses not to control his or her problem when there is a good chance that he or she could.

To these unfortunate psoriatics, I say turn the tide by making those around you the center of *your* concern. Who knows? Such a thoughtful act may, in itself, lead to a miracle. In other words, it is the patient who is doing something for somebody else.

*Group IV.* They will combine the efforts of Edgar Cayce and ortho-dox medicine, which could bring about incredible results. As soon as possible, however, they should lean more toward the natural alternative and avoid medical interventions that may have serious side effects.

*Group V.* They usually revert back to orthodox management if it is their nature to be totally undisciplined. In extreme cases, this can mean a series of hospital stays for the rest of their lives.

The patient, you see, has to *decide* what is most important to him. Does he really want to get rid of the disease or doesn't he? Is the effort to change his lifestyle really worth it? This must be determined, for the decision will strongly influence the final outcome.

In all fairness, it has been my experience that the vast major-ity of patients do truly wish to be healed. This attitude makes all the years of study, effort, experimentation, and risk worth the price. If the treatment is successful, the patient is always delighted, but as a physician, I can think of no greater reward than the joy, the glow of happiness, the sense of accomplish-ment, that comes with the knowledge that my patient is well!

## To Sum Up

With this book, I have endeavored to lay before you my efforts, span-ning more than thirty-five years, to solve the riddle of psoriasis. My research suggests that psoriasis is a symptom with a deeper underlying cause. Treat the symptoms only, and you will forever have psoriasis; treat the cause, and it is possible to rid yourself, or at least have control, of the disease forever.

The external manifestation (the lesions) is the result of an overabundant toxic accumulation within the system being expelled through the sweat glands. The toxic accumulation in the lymph and blood is due principally to intestinal permeability (leaky gut). The alleviation, control, healing, and regeneration of the surface cells (your skin) depend on two factors, primarily: (1) ensuring adequate drainage of toxins through the normal channels of elimination, namely your bowels and kidneys, and (2) not polluting the body further by ingesting elements destructive to the gut wall, achieved by following a carefully selective diet. All other suggestions within the Cayce/Pagano regimen are aids to this healing process. When these factors, combined with patience and persistence, are put into motion for a long enough period of time, the end result can be a healing of the intestinal walls followed by a complete disappearance of all lesions, anywhere and everywhere.

This book offers a choice to the patient. He or she can embrace the information presented here or ignore it. The future of the patient depends on the choice made. I have done my best to present my case in such a way that the patient chooses wisely. I can do no more—the rest is up to you. But, in choosing the course to follow, remember to have faith in the power of your own mind. The thoughts you choose each day have a direct influence on your state of health.

Dada J. P. Vaswani, a beloved spiritual teacher of India, declared, "Thoughts are the building blocks of life. With thoughts we are building our own future." And as Edgar Cayce repeatedly emphasized, "Thoughts are things!"

> So my dear reader, do not despair,
> Keep your spirits high,
> For there is more to you, indeed
> Than meets the naked eye!

# APPENDIX A

# Nutritional Considerations in the Natural Healing of Psoriasis, Eczema, and Psoriatic Arthritis

Approval by your personal physician is essential before embarking on this or any other dietary program. Avoid any food item that causes an allergic reaction, even if it is on the permitted list.

## The 80 Percent–20 Percent Food Ratio

*Eighty percent* of the daily food intake should be selected from the following list, most of which are alkaline (base) formers:

*Water:* Six to eight glasses of pure water daily in addition to all other liquids consumed

*Lecithin:* Granular—1 tablespoon three times per day, five days per week

*Fruit:* Fresh is preferred, frozen is permitted, packed in water in glass jars on occasion. Stewed fruits are highly recommended, whenever possible.

*Allowed:* Apples (cooked), apricots, most berries, cherries, dates, figs (unsulphured), grapefruit, grapes, kiwis, lemons, limes, mangoes, nectarines, oranges, papayas, peaches, pears, pineapples, and small prunes.

*Permitted in lesser quantities:* Avocados, cranberries, currants, plums and large prunes. Note that raw apples, bananas, and melons are permitted provided they are eaten alone and sparingly.

(No strawberries or citrus fruits are allowed in cases of eczema or arthritis, and no strawberries in cases of psoriasis.)

*Vegetables:* Daily intake should be three that grow above the ground to one that grows below the ground. Fresh is preferred, frozen is permitted, packed in glass jars on occasion.

> *Allowed:* Asparagus, beets, broccoli, Brussels sprouts, cabbage, carrots*, celery*, cucumbers, garlic*, lettuce* (romaine in particular), onions*, olives, parsnips, pumpkin, scallions, soybeans, spinach*, sprouts*, string beans, squash, sweet potatoes, watercress*. (Note: Those marked with an asterisk are particularly important.)

> *Permitted in lesser quantities:* Corn (white corn is preferred), dried beans, lentils, mushrooms, peas, and rhubarb.

*Juices:* Daily intake of freshly made vegetable and fruit juice is highly recommended. The most valuable kitchen appliance investment is a juicer or a blender. Most effective is one glass per day of freshly juiced carrots, celery, and lettuce.

*Miscellaneous:* Almonds are alkaline in nature. Eating five raw almonds a day is suggested. Filberts are permitted occasionally as well as chestnuts and fresh coconut. Apple cider vinegar (used sparingly) is the only type of vinegar permitted.

*Twenty percent* of the daily food intake should be selected from the following, most of which are acid formers:

*Grains:* Most grains are acid formers (except millet) and should be consumed in the form of natural whole-grain products such as bagels, breads, cereals (with very little, if any, preservatives or artificial sweeteners), muffins, pasta (Jerusalem artichoke is preferred, with olive oil and garlic sauce), rice (brown and/or wild is preferred)—no white-flour products.

*Meats:*

> Fish—fresh or frozen salt- or freshwater, white-fleshed varieties are permitted, but dark, oily is preferred (no shellfish). If canned, water or oil packed is permitted. Fish is suggested about three to four times per week.

> Poultry—chicken, Cornish hen, turkey, wild fowl (all skinless, white meat is preferred). Poultry is permitted about two or three times per week.

Lamb—trimmed of all fat before cooking, well done, once or twice a week (never fried, and no more than 4 to 6 ounces at a serving).

*Dairy:* Only low-fat/low-sodium products are permitted: skim, low-fat, 1% or 2% milk, cheese, buttermilk, yogurt, and so forth (no ice cream, cream toppings, or whole-milk products). Dairy products, for the most part, are classified as being neutral or alkaline in their reaction, depending on the source of reference. Do not have citrus fruits or citrus juices with dairy products or cereals at the same meal.

*Butter:* Regular butter is permitted, but only occasionally and very sparingly. (Even though it is a saturated fat, a little butter is better than margarine and other hydrogenated products.)

*Eggs:* Two to four per week, prepared any way except fried.

*Oils:* Canola, coconut, corn, cottonseed, olive, safflower, sesame, soybean, sunflower, and occasionally peanut. One teaspoon of olive oil three times per day is suggested for children, and one tablespoon three times per day for adults, unless there is a gallbladder problem.

*Teas:* Slippery elm bark powder (in the morning) and American yellow saffron (in the evening) as directed are the teas most beneficial in psoriasis and eczema cases. (Chamomile, green, mullein, oolong, or watermelon seed tea may be substituted at times for the American yellow saffron tea.) Remember, pregnant women or those anticipating pregnancy should avoid both the slippery elm and saffron teas.

## Foods to Avoid

*Almost all saturated fats:* Red meats (except lamb) such as beef, pork, sweetbreads, and veal; processed meats such as bologna, pepperoni, frankfurters, salami, and sausage; hydrogenated products such as margarine and shortening. Avoid trans fats as much as possible.

*The nightshades:* Eggplant, paprika, peppers (all types except black pepper), tomatoes (and tomato sauces and products), tobacco (smoking), white potatoes (all potatoes are considered "white" except sweet potatoes and yams).

*Shellfish:* Clams, crabs, lobster, shrimp, and sauces made with shellfish.

*Junk food:* Candy and pastries, chocolate (and all products made with chocolate, including white chocolate), french fries, potato chips, soda (diet and regular), and sweets. These junk foods are a major cause of psoriasis and eczema in adults as well as children.

*Yeast:* Or yeast-laden foods, if there is an underlying yeast infection (candidiasis).

*Coffee:* If strongly desired, a maximum of three cups per day of black decaffeinated coffee may be consumed. Remember, coffee is a diuretic, and if taken too often, it depletes calcium from the body, especially after age forty. Therefore, replace the calcium by having one or two cups of skim milk or other foods that supply calcium at a different time of the day. It is best not to mix milk or sugar into coffee.

*Gluten:* And products containing gluten, such as barley, oats, rye, and wheat, if allergies or celiac disease is suspected.

*Miscellaneous:* All fried foods, pizza, alcohol (including beer), sugary cereals, vinegar (wine or grain), pickled and smoked foods, hot spices, gravies, strawberries, peanut butter, and too many starches.

*Note:* In every case of psoriatic arthritis and eczema, avoid citrus fruits, citrus juices, strawberries, and adding salt to foods. Added salt in general should be avoided. The salt (sodium) found naturally in the daily diet is quite adequate for most people.

## Above- and Below-Ground Vegetables

Most vegetables, as well as fruits, are alkaline formers and purifiers of the blood. Vegetables should be chosen and consumed on a daily basis in these proportions: three that grow above the ground to one that grows below the ground. Examples of above- and below-ground vegetables follow (prohibited vegetables have been omitted):

**Above Ground (Choose three)**

| | |
|---|---|
| Artichokes | Cucumber |
| Asparagus | Dandelion greens |
| Beans (including soybeans, lentils, peas) | Endive |
| | Fennel |
| Broccoli | Leeks |
| Brussels sprouts | Lettuce (all types) |
| Cabbage | Olives |
| Cauliflower | Parsley |
| Celery | Pumpkin |
| Chicory | Spinach |
| Chives | Watercress |
| | Zucchini |

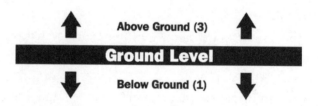

**Below Ground (Choose one)**

| | |
|---|---|
| Beets | Parsnips |
| Carrots | Salsify (oyster plant) |
| Garlic | Radishes |
| Jerusalem artichoke (sunchoke) | Sweet potatoes |
| | Turnips |
| Onions | Yams |

*Note:* Onions, lettuce, celery, spinach, and carrots, are particularly recommended.

## Proteins and Starches

The following list contains proteins and starches that are permitted in the diet, but these should not be combined to too great an extent with one another at the same meal.

**Proteins**

All types of grains

Avocados

Cheese

Dried beans, peas, soybeans and lentils

Eggs

Fish, fowl, and lamb

Milk

Nuts

Olives

**Starches**

All cereals

Beets, burdock, carrots, parsnips, rutabaga, salsify (oyster plant), water chestnuts (all alkaline reacting)

Bran

Breads and crackers

Corn and rice

Dried beans and peas

Grains: barley, buckwheat, millet, oats, rye, and so forth

Squash (winter), pumpkin, and yams

Syrups and sugars (use only those permitted)

*Note:* Some items are listed under both categories because they are a protein as well as a starch.

# Principles of Breakfast, Lunch, and Dinner

Remember, each meal is important; do not skip meals.

## Suggested Breakfast Meals

The slippery elm tea should be taken at least a half hour before breakfast for best results, unless it was taken the night before.

Most breakfast foods in the American diet are largely acid formers and should therefore not be consumed in very large portions. Foods such as whole-grain cereals (hot or cold), breads, muffins, pancakes, and so forth, are acid forming. Other, desirable breakfast foods such as stewed fruits, baked apples, stewed figs, and stewed apricots are alkaline forming.

Hot cereals should not be cooked too long, as this destroys the vitamins and minerals necessary for building greater resistance in the body. Any noncitrus fruit, chopped or slivered almonds, or a little honey or pure maple syrup may be added to hot or cold cereal.

Citrus fruits and citrus fruit juices (primarily orange and grapefruit) must not be eaten at the same meal with cereals, gruels, or dairy products. Citrus fruits may be eaten alone, unless the patient experiences a reaction such as itching, rash, or hypersensitivity of any kind. If this occurs, I advise my patients to curtail or eliminate citrus from their diet altogether, at least temporarily.

The most desirable fruit juices are those of the noncitrus variety such as apricot, pear, grape, apple, mango, papaya, and the like. (Cranberry is acid forming.)

Keep in mind that raw apples, bananas, and melons, although permitted on the diet, should be eaten by themselves as a snack between meals, not eaten at meals with other foods.

Eggs (two to four per week) are permitted, unless the patient is on a special low-cholesterol diet. They may be boiled (preferably soft boiled or coddled), steamed, or cooked in a nonstick pan without oil or fat of any kind.

Milk; cheese; yogurt with active cultures is highly suggested; buttermilk; and so forth should always be of the low-fat (or nonfat), low-salt variety. Skim milk and products made with skim milk are preferred.

Black decaffeinated coffee is permitted (no cream or sugar), but no more than three cups per day. Some patients substitute a cup of hot water with the juice of a fresh lemon in the morning in place of coffee.

Jelly preserves, 100 percent pure, without preservatives or additives, may be spread lightly on whole-grain toast or English muffins as a substitute for butter or margarine.

While these rules may seem challenging to many patients, once they get the idea, the rules become second nature to them, and the patients proceed without difficulty.

## Suggested Lunch Meals

Lunch should consist primarily of fresh, raw, green leafy vegetables, especially celery, spinach, watercress, and all types of lettuce, particularly romaine, at least four times a week. Olive oil combined with fresh lemon juice is the preferred salad dressing. Ingredients such as a little water or oil packed white albacore tuna, sliced white-meat turkey or chicken breast, hard-boiled eggs, tofu, feta, low-fat cottage cheese, and other types of salt-free, low-fat cheese may be added on occasion for variety. A good alternate is a fresh fruit salad. A cup of homemade fat-free soup or broth may be included as part of lunch, if desired.

Freshly grated or finely chopped vegetables such as carrots, celery, beets, watercress, and so forth, combined in gelatin and served on a bed of green leafy vegetables, is also highly recommended, as are fresh fruits and their juices in gelatin. The nutrients in these foods are absorbed and assimilated by the body to a much greater degree when combined with gelatin. These particular types of salads may be chosen as a luncheon meal or eaten as a snack at any time. Vegetarians may use agar agar in place of animal-based gelatin.

## Suggested Dinner Meals

Dinner should consist of a raw vegetable salad, at least two or three cooked vegetables, and no more than a six-ounce portion of fish, lamb, or poultry. Vegetables cooked in Patapar or vegetable parchment paper are baked in their own juices and thereby retain all their vital nutrients. This method of cooking vegetables is preferred above all others; however, vegetables may also be steamed, baked, microwaved, pressure cooked, or stir-fried. (*Note:* Stir-frying does not mean frying foods in large amounts of oil or fat, but is rather the Asian method of quickly cooking diced, chopped, or shredded foods such as meats, fish, chicken, turkey, or vegetables in a wok or heavy skillet for a few minutes, or until tender, in very little oil.) Shortening and refined fats and oils (unsaturated as well as saturated) should never be used when cooking foods. It is best not to overcook vegetables or deep-fry them.

# Food Combinations to Avoid

Most people are not aware that certain foods should not be combined at the same meal although they may be eaten separately. This is because some food combinations may cause havoc within the body, sooner or later showing their deleterious effect in the form of poor digestion, as well as improper utilization and assimilation of vital nutrients. When this occurs, the end result is intestinal discomfort, malnutrition, and poor elimination. Add the overabundance of acid formers, and you have the breeding ground for a generalized toxic buildup. For these reasons, the following food combinations are to be avoided. When preparing meals, the proper 80 percent alkaline–20 percent acid ratio should always be kept in mind.

- Do not combine whole-grain products such as cereals, breads, and so forth with citrus fruits, citrus juices, or stewed or dried fruits.
- Do not combine citrus fruits or their juices with dairy products such as cheese, milk, or yogurt.
- Do not combine any type of fruit with white-flour products such as bread, crackers, cereals, pasta, and so forth.
- Do not combine melons (any variety), raw apples, or bananas with other foods. These fruits may, however, be eaten separately.
- Do not combine milk, cream, or sugar with coffee or tea.
- Do not combine too many acid-forming foods (proteins, starches, sugars, fats and oils) at the same meal.

# Reminders

- The suggested amount of water intake, six to eight glasses of pure water daily, is in addition to all other beverages (juice, tea, coffee, and so forth).
- Granular lecithin may be added to beverages or sprinkled on foods.
- Herbal teas are best consumed without adding milk, cream, or sugar. Leave them pure.

- It is best to drink American yellow saffron tea more often than the other suggested herbal teas. However, it should not be consumed too soon after taking slippery elm tea. A time lapse of several hours between drinking these particular teas is suggested. (Avoid these teas if you are pregnant or plan to become pregnant.)

- A maximum of 3 cups of naturally decaffeinated coffee is permitted per day. Milk, cream, or sugar should not be added.

- The primary cleansers of the body are fruit and fruit juices, pure water, and the herbal teas. The primary builders of the body are vegetables and vegetable juices. These cleansers and builders are the mainstay of the diet. The relatively few fruits and vegetables that are acid-forming need not be of too much concern, unless a decided adverse reaction occurs. If this happens, they should be avoided. Learn how to listen to your own body.

- Between-meal snacks are optional.

- Always choose foods carefully when preparing a daily or weekly menu. Try to vary your selection of foods to prevent a feeling of deprivation or boredom.

- It is best to use sparing amounts of spices, sweeteners, butter, and oils when cooking or adding to foods.

- Blood cholesterol and acid levels are reduced by limiting fat and sugar intake.

- Foods that cause an allergic reaction should be avoided even if they appear on the permitted food list.

- Carbonated drinks, especially regular and diet soda, are not permitted. The only exception is seltzer (not club soda) or naturally carbonated spring waters, to which may be added lemon or lime juice. Even these beverages should be consumed only on an occasional basis.

- Fresh fruits, vegetables, and high-fiber foods are the best sources of maintaining adequate, daily bowel movements. In addition to these foods, home enemas or natural cathartics often aid in cases of chronic constipation. High-colonic irrigations should be professionally administered and only with the approval of a licensed physician.

- Red or white wine (2 to 4 ounces) may be consumed occasionally if you are not on any medication or suffering from gout.
- All dairy products such as milk, cheese, and yogurt should be skim or low-fat varieties and consumed only in moderate amounts.
- A good substitute for a cup of coffee is a cup of hot water flavored with lemon or lime juice.
- Overeating is never advocated, even with the foods that are allowed. Eat less, live longer!

To purchase *Dr. John's Healing Psoriasis Cookbook . . . Plus!,* which contains more than three hundred recipes designed for the psoriasis, eczema, and psoriatic-arthritis patient, visit my Web site, www.psoriasis-healing .com, or call 201-947-0606.

# APPENDIX B

# Menu Plans and Recipes

## Dr. John's Seven-Day Sample Menu Plan

Recipes marked with an asterisk (*) are taken from *Dr. John's Healing Psoriasis Cookbook . . . Plus!* Recipes marked with two asterisks (**) were created for this edition by Marjorie May. *Note:* If you feel you are losing too much weight, double up on the permitted foods. Avoid any foods you know you are allergic to.

## Day 1

### Breakfast
- Stewed figs
- Oatmeal-Cinnamon Hotcakes**
- Hot lemon water, herbal tea, or black decaffeinated coffee

### Lunch
- Tofu and Spinach Soup*
- Charlton Tuna Salad*
- Shredded lettuce and carrots on the side
- Herbal tea, lemon water, or spring or filtered water

### Dinner
- Broiled Lamb Patties with Marinade**
- Deluxe Acorn Squash**
- Green salad with at least three to four varieties of greens
- Sugar-free Jell-O with a small dollop of whipped cream
- Herbal tea, lemon water, or spring or filtered water

283

Between meal snack suggestions: See the permitted list following this menu. Follow the list of daily suggestions found at the end of the Seven-Day Sample Menu Plan.

## Day 2

### Breakfast

- Bowl of oatmeal topped with sliced almonds if desired (optional: add 1 teaspoon olive oil for children, or 1 tablespoon for adults)
- ½ cup low-fat or skim milk or unsweetened soy milk
- ½ cup stewed apples with cinnamon, sweetened with Splenda or stevia if desired
- Hot lemon water, herbal tea, or black decaffeinated coffee

### Lunch

- Green Goddess Soup**
- Oriental Chicken Salad*
- Bunch white grapes or sliced pear or apricot
- Herbal tea, lemon water, or spring or filtered water

### Dinner

- Salmon—grilled, baked, or poached
- Steamed asparagus (drizzled with olive oil and/or tiny pat of butter if desired)
- Mixed-greens salad with shredded carrots and cut-up squash
- Oranges and unsweetened pineapple chunks or unsweetened yogurt
- Herbal tea, lemon water, or spring or filtered water

## Day 3

### Breakfast

- One or two brown rice (or buckwheat) waffles toasted (found in frozen food section in supermarkets and health food stores). Add olive oil to taste and a sprinkle of cinnamon and a small drizzle of honey if desired.
- One or two scrambled eggs (use 1 egg yolk to 2 egg whites)
- Fresh or frozen cherries or blueberries
- Hot lemon water, herbal tea, or black decaffeinated coffee

## Lunch

- Cup of tomato-free veggie broth (read ingredient labels)
- Turkey burger grilled or broiled, with onions and/or leek or chopped garlic sautéed in grapeseed or canola oil
- Slice of spelt or millet bread
- Mixed-greens salad with herb dressing or lemon juice and olive oil
- Herbal tea, lemon water, or spring or filtered water

## Dinner

- Poached Orange Roughy with Spinach*
- Roasted Carrots and Parsnips*
- Coleslaw*
- 1 cup sliced pears and/or applesauce
- Herbal tea, lemon water, or spring or filtered water

# Day 4

## Breakfast

- Permitted dry cereal (preferred are amaranth, millet, or quinoa)
- Low-fat, skim, or soy milk
- ½ cup lowfat plain yogurt or stewed apricots or pears
- Hot lemon water, herbal tea, or black decaffeinated coffee

## Lunch

- Chunk white tuna with mixed-greens salad topped with Italian dressing
- Vegetable broth—add leftover veggies or low-carb pasta if desired or available
- Spring water or herbal tea

## Dinner

- Chicken—cut, marinate one hour in 2 tablespoons Italian dressing; bake at 375 degrees Fahrenheit for forty minutes
- Baked sweet potato, seasoned with olive oil or strained yogurt with fresh or dried chives added

- Steamed peas with pearl onions seasoned with olive oil and/or small pat of butter
- Spring water or herbal tea

## Day 5

### Breakfast

- Two scrambled egg whites and one egg yolk, whipped with 2 tablespoons milk or sugar-free soy milk
- One whole-grain English muffin with olive oil and/or a dab of butter and/or unsweetened preserves
- Hot lemon water, herbal tea, or black decaffeinated coffee

### Lunch

- Tofu and Spinach Soup*
- Brown Rice with Lentils*
- Cut-up broccoli and pine nuts tossed with Barbara's Broccoli Dip*
- Spring water or herbal tea

### Dinner

- Green Vegetable Casserole*
- Broiled Flounder Fillets* or any desired fish
- Carrot and celery sticks
- Spring water or herbal tea

## Day 6

### Breakfast

- One or two poached eggs
- One or two slices spelt toast topped with olive oil
- Fresh or frozen raspberries or blueberries
- Hot lemon water, herbal tea, or black decaffeinated coffee

### Lunch

- Apple–Butternut Squash Soup*
- Cold Tuna-Noodle Salad*

- Fresh sliced bok choy and/or celery sticks
- Spring water or herbal tea

### Dinner
- Roast Turkey Breast*
- Sesame Noodles with Kale*
- Fresh cucumber slices
- Spring water or herbal tea

## Day 7
### Breakfast
- Cream of Wheat cereal with sliced almonds and honey if desired
- ½ cup skim milk or low-fat, no-sugar soy milk (such as Edensoy)
- Stewed apples sweetened with honey and cinnamon
- Hot lemon water, herbal tea, or black decaffeinated coffee

### Lunch
- Chicken and Zucchini Soup*
- Garbanzo Bean Salad*
- Sliced leftover turkey on a bed of romaine lettuce with mixed raw permitted veggies
- Spring water or herbal tea

### Dinner
- Baked Fish à la Dee*
- Brown rice simmered in chicken broth
- Fresh mixed-greens salad with Lemon Vinaigrette Dressing*
- 1 small piece Aunt Tina's Honey Carrot Cake*
- Spring water or herbal tea

## Daily Suggestions—for Every Day
- Six to eight glasses of spring or filtered water. (It is best to drink water or other liquids thirty minutes before or after meals but not during.)

- Herbal teas: Slippery elm bark powder and American yellow saffron. (*Caution:* These should not be taken if you are pregnant or anticipating pregnancy.)
- A few raw almonds.
- Three tablespoons of olive oil (for children: 3 teaspoons).
- A medium to large mixed-greens salad without nightshades, unless there is an underlying irritable bowel condition, in which case green leafy salads would be contraindicated.
- There should be a complete evacuation of the bowels one to three times per day.
- One to three tablespoons of granular lecithin in water or sprinkled on any appropriate food (for children 1 to 3 teaspoons)—unless there is an allergy to soy.
- Permitted proteins (prepared any way but fried or smoked): Lamb (well-done, all fat removed, once per week); chicken, turkey, wild game (may be cooked with the skin on, but do not eat the skin—twice per week); fish (the most valuable animal protein, contains omega-3, four times per week).

## Permitted List of Between-Meal Snacks

- Raw apples, banana, grapes
- Celery and carrot sticks
- Bowl of cut-up melon
- Bowl of blueberries and cut-up mango
- Plain yogurt (with active cultures)
- Five to twelve raw almonds
- Ricotta cheese or almond butter spread on one slice whole-grain bread or four to five whole-grain crackers
- Hard-boiled egg with one slice whole-grain toast topped with olive oil
- Whole-grain English muffin with melted white, hard cheese, such as Swiss

# The Recipes

Recipes are in the same order as they appear in the sample menu plan. Note that organic foods should be used whenever possible. Most stores carry organic produce and breads. The Whole Foods chain, if available to you, carries organic foods in almost all categories. Many large supermarkets are now carrying many organic foods. If organic foods are not available, ask the store manager to stock them. Remember, just because an item says "natural" does not mean it is organic. Certified organic foods are produced without pesticides, artificial fertilizers, GMOs, and, in the case of dairy, no hormones. Eating primarily organic foods will help further to eliminate toxins from the body. If you cannot find organic foods, do the best you can and try to drink a little more pure water to flush out any extra toxins in your system.

## OATMEAL-CINNAMON HOTCAKES—WITH VARIATIONS
### Serves 2 (halve ingredients to serve 1; double to serve 4)

1 cup oatmeal
½ teaspoon baking soda
¼ teaspoon salt
1 teaspoon ground cinnamon
½ teaspoon honey

2 tablespoons grapeseed oil, plus extra for coating skillet
1 egg
⅓ cup milk
¼-inch pieces

1. Pour the oatmeal, baking soda, salt, and cinnamon into a blender or Magic Bullet (a handy appliance for small blending jobs) and blend until flourlike in consistency. Put this mixture into a bowl.
2. Place the honey, oil, egg, and milk into the blender or Magic Bullet and mix well.
3. Pour the wet mixture into the dry mixture in the bowl and stir with a spoon until evenly mixed.
4. Coat a skillet lightly with grapeseed oil and heat to medium-hot.
5. Pour the mixture into the hot skillet, making two large round hotcakes or four smaller ones. Cook until golden and then flip and cook until golden on the other side.
6. Top with warmed sugar-free applesauce and cinnamon, if desired, or with 1 tablespoon olive oil, warmed, or ½ pat butter per serving, and cinnamon to taste.

*Variations*

**Oatmeal-Apple-Cinnamon Hotcakes**

Follow the directions for Oatmeal-Cinnamon Hotcakes. Stir ¼ cup finely diced apples into the mixture just before pouring into the skillet. Continue cooking the hotcakes as directed.

**Oatmeal-Blueberry Hotcakes**

Follow the directions for Oatmeal-Cinnamon Hotcakes. Just before pouring the mixture into the skillet, mix in ¼ cup of fresh blueberries. Continue cooking the hotcakes as directed.

## TOFU AND SPINACH SOUP
*Serves 6*

8 cups water
½ cup chopped onions
1–1½ teaspoons Superior Touch "Better than Bouillon" (vegetable or chicken base), or 1–1½ cubes chicken or vegetable bouillon

1 (12-ounce) package tofu (firm or extra-firm), diced
2–3 cups fresh spinach cut into strips (or use frozen chopped spinach)
Ground black pepper (optional)

1. Bring the water to a boil in a saucepan, then add the onions.
2. Cook until the onions are done, then add the bouillon and return to a boil.
3. Add the tofu and spinach, bring to a boil again. Add ground black pepper, if desired.

## CHARLTON TUNA SALAD
*Serves 1*

1 (6-ounce) can tuna in water, drained and flaked
½ cup low-fat or nonfat plain yogurt
1 teaspoon dried dill
1 teaspoon dried mint

¼ teaspoon black pepper
4 lettuce leaves
¼ pound white seedless grapes, divided, for garnish
2 slices lemon, for garnish

1. In a medium bowl, mix together the tuna, yogurt, herbs, and pepper. Cover and chill for 1 hour.
2. To serve, place on the lettuce leaves and garnish with the grapes and lemon. Serve with a whole-grain roll, if desired.

## BROILED LAMB PATTIES WITH MARINADE
*Serves 2*

1 pound ground lamb (organic if available)
¼ cup celery, finely chopped
¼ cup onion, finely chopped

1 teaspoon California ground, dried garlic and parsley
½ teaspoon sea salt
¼ cup zesty Italian dressing

1. Early in the day, mix together the lamb, celery, onion, garlic/parsley, and sea salt. Form into patties.
2. Place in a resealable plastic bag with the zesty Italian dressing and shake gently so as not to break up the patties. Store in the refrigerator, shaking occasionally, until ready to broil.
3. Preheat the broiler.
4. Place the lamb patties on the rack over the broiling pan. Broil about 2 inches from the heat source.
5. Broil for 8 minutes, turning once, or until the patties are well done.

## DELUXE ACORN SQUASH
*Serves 2*

1 large acorn squash
½ teaspoon salt, or to taste
2 tablespoons canola or grapeseed oil
¼ teaspoon butter

¼–½ teaspoon Splenda or stevia or honey
1 teaspoon cinnamon, or to taste

1. Cut up the squash and steam until soft.
2. Mash the squash, then add the remaining ingredients, mixing until well combined.

## GREEN GODDESS SOUP (ADAPTED FROM DR. JOHN'S JUNGLE BREW)
### Serves 4

1 tablespoon butter
1 tablespoon olive oil
1 large sweet onion, coarsely chopped
1 leek, sliced into ½-inch pieces, some of green part included
3 stalks celery, stringy part removed, cut into 2-inch pieces
1 Jerusalem artichoke (sunchoke), pared and thinly sliced (optional)

2 sprigs fresh parsley, stems removed, coarsely chopped
1½ cups water
3 ounces spinach, washed well
½ head romaine lettuce
½ cup soy milk (optional, if creamy texture is desired)
Salt and pepper (optional)

1. In a large pot, combine the butter, olive oil, onion, leek, celery, Jerusalem artichoke, and parsley. Sauté lightly, stirring, until the vegetables begin to soften and turn golden. Add ½ cup of the water and simmer for 10 minutes. Place in a blender and puree until smooth. Return to the pot and set aside.
2. Pour the remaining 1 cup of water into the blender. Gradually add the spinach and lettuce. Puree until smooth. Pour the pureed lettuce mixture into the pot containing the other vegetables. Stir to mix. Simmer for 5 more minutes.
3. Optional: If a creamier texture is desired, add the soy milk, salt, and pepper to taste. Reheat as desired.

## ORIENTAL CHICKEN SALAD
### Serves 6 to 8

2½ cups broccoli florets, steamed until crisp
1 cup fresh mushrooms, sliced
1 cup snow pea pods, cleaned

½ cup scallions, chopped
1 pound grilled chicken breast, cut into chunks

### Dressing

¼ cup olive oil
2 teaspoons sesame oil
1 tablespoon fresh lemon juice
1 tablespoon fresh dill, chopped

3–4 garlic cloves, minced
½ teaspoon salt
½ teaspoon pepper

1. Mix all of the dressing ingredients in a bowl until well blended. Set aside.
2. In a large bowl, mix together the broccoli, mushrooms, snow pea pods, and scallions. Add the dressing, then chill for a couple of hours.
3. Just before eating, add the chicken chunks, toss, and serve.

## POACHED ORANGE ROUGHY WITH SPINACH
### Serves 4

2 packages frozen spinach leaves
1½ pounds orange roughy
¾ cup water
¼ cup dry white wine

⅛ teaspoon dried thyme
½ teaspoon dried parsley flakes
2 tablespoons red onions, chopped
pepper

1. Cook the spinach according to the package directions and set aside.
2. Cut the fish into 4 to 6-ounce serving-size portions and set aside.
3. Combine the remaining ingredients in a large nonstick skillet and bring to a boil. Add the fish and return to a boil. Lower the heat, cover, and simmer gently for about 6 minutes.
4. When ready to serve, put some spinach on each serving plate. Remove the fish with a slotted spatula and place on the spinach. Spoon some of the cooking juices over the fish and spinach.

*Note:* You may substitute white fish or sea bass fillets for the orange roughy in this recipe.

## ROASTED CARROTS AND PARSNIPS
### Serves 6

2 pounds parsnips
1 pound carrots
3 tablespoons olive oil

½ teaspoon dried rosemary
sea salt and black pepper

1. Preheat oven to 375°F.
2. Peel the parsnips and carrots and cut into ¾-inch slices. In a large bowl, toss the vegetables together with the oil and rosemary.
3. Spread in a single layer in a shallow baking dish and season with salt and pepper. You may need to use two baking dishes if one is not large enough.
4. Roast the vegetables in the oven, stirring occasionally, until brown and crisp, about 25 minutes.

## COLESLAW
### Serves 4 to 6

¼ cup fresh parsley
½ small onion
1 carrot, cut into 1-inch pieces or shredded
1 cabbage (about 2 pounds)

½ cup low-fat mayonnaise
½ cup low-fat yogurt
pinch of fructose
2 tablespoons apple cider vinegar
sea salt and pepper

1. In a food processor with the metal blade in place, combine the parsley, onion, and carrot. Process, turning the machine on and off until they are finely minced. Empty into a large bowl.
2. Insert the slicing disk into the food processor. Cut the cabbage into wedges to fit the tube. Place a wedge into the tube and process, using light pressure, almost letting the cabbage go through by itself. Add to the vegetables in the bowl. Repeat with the remaining cabbage.
3. Add the rest of the ingredients to the bowl and mix well. Adjust the seasoning and refrigerate.
*Note:* You can cut all vegetables by hand, using a sharp knife.

## BROWN RICE WITH LENTILS
### Serves 4 to 6

3 tablespoons safflower oil
1 large onion, chopped
2 cups uncooked brown rice

½ cup brown lentils
4 cups boiling water
sea salt

1. In a heavy, deep pan, heat the oil, add the onions, and sauté until transparent and lightly flecked with brown. Add the rice and lentils and stir over medium heat for 3 minutes.
2. Add the boiling water slowly and salt to taste. Return to a boil, stirring occasionally. Lower the heat, cover, and simmer gently for 45 minutes, or until the liquid is absorbed.
3. Remove from the heat and let stand for 10 to 15 minutes before serving.

### BARBARA'S BROCCOLI DIP
*Serves 6 to 8*

| | |
|---|---|
| 1 bunch broccoli stems, peeled and cut into chunks | 2 cups low-fat mayonnaise |
| 4 scallions | 2 tablespoons extra-virgin olive oil |
| 8–10 sprigs fresh parsley | 1 teaspoon lemon juice |
| 6–8 sprigs fresh dill | ½ teaspoon sea salt |
| | ¼ teaspoon black pepper |

1. Place all of the vegetables and herbs in a food processor. Process for several minutes until finely chopped.
2. Add the remaining ingredients and mix well. Chill for two hours before serving. May be kept for several days in the refrigerator.

### GREEN VEGETABLE CASSEROLE
*Serves 3 to 4*

| | |
|---|---|
| 2 cups leeks, finely chopped | 1 cup scallions, finely chopped |
| 2 cups spinach, finely chopped | 1½ tablespoons all-purpose flour |
| 1 cup romaine lettuce, finely chopped | 1 teaspoon sea salt |
| 1 cup fresh parsley, finely chopped | ½ teaspoon black pepper |
| | 8 eggs |
| | 1 tablespoon olive oil |

1. Preheat the oven to 325°F.
2. Place all of the chopped vegetables in a large bowl and mix well. Add the flour, salt, and pepper, and mix well.
3. In another bowl, beat the eggs and add them to the vegetables. Mix well.

4. Rub the inside of a rectangular glass baking dish with the olive oil. Pour the vegetable mixture into the dish. Bake for an hour, or until the top is crisp and browned. May be served hot or cold. This dish is delicious served with plain yogurt.

## BROILED FLOUNDER FILLETS
### Serves 4

6 flounder fillets, washed and patted dry
white pepper
1 tablespoon corn oil
2 tablespoons low-fat mayonnaise

1 tablespoon Dijon mustard
1 teaspoon fresh lemon juice
¼ teaspoon dried parsley flakes
4 lemon wedges

1. Preheat the broiler to high.
2. Place flounder fillets on a flat surface. Sprinkle with the pepper and brush with the oil.
3. In a bowl, blend the mayonnaise, mustard, lemon juice, and parsley. Brush evenly over the fish.
4. Place the fish under the broiler, 3 to 4 inches from the source of heat. Broil for 4 to 5 minutes, or until golden brown and the fish is just cooked through. Serve with lemon wedges.

## COLD TUNA-NOODLE SALAD
### Serves 4 to 6

1 (8-ounce) box DeBoles Jerusalem Artichoke Pasta (any shape)
2 tablespoons olive oil
1 (6-ounce) can white albacore tuna in water, drained
2 tablespoons low-cholesterol mayonnaise

1 medium-size red onion, diced
2 hard-boiled eggs, cooled and chopped coarsely
salt and pepper (optional)
Any permitted vegetable (such as carrots, broccoli, celery), diced (optional)

1. Cook the pasta per the package directions. Drain and stir in the olive oil. Let cool.
2. Add the remaining ingredients and mix well. Serve chilled. (You could also serve it warm—it's delicious either way!)

## APPLE AND BUTTERNUT SQUASH SOUP
### Serves 8

1 pound butternut squash
3 medium-size tart apples
1 medium-size onion
1 stalk celery
¼ teaspoon dried rosemary
¼ teaspoon dried marjoram
3 (14½-ounce) cans low-fat,
   low-salt chicken broth

1 cup water
1 teaspoon sea salt
¼ teaspoon black pepper
3 tablespoons fresh parsley,
   chopped, for garnish

1. Cut the squash in half, and seed, peel, and dice it. Do the same for the apples. Peel and roughly chop the onion and celery.
2. Place all of the ingredients except the parsley in a large stockpot. Over high heat, bring to a boil. Lower the heat and simmer for 45 minutes.
3. With a slotted spoon, remove the squash and apples and place in a blender or food processor. Purée until smooth. Add back to the stock and stir. Garnish with the parsley.

*Note:* This soup may be frozen.

## ROAST TURKEY BREAST
### Serves 8 to 10

½ teaspoon poultry seasoning
¼ teaspoon dried thyme
2 tablespoons olive oil

pinch of sea salt and pepper
1 (6–7 pound) turkey breast

1. Preheat the oven to 325°F. Mix together all of the ingredients except the turkey. Brush this mixture all over the turkey breast.
2. Place the turkey breast skin side up on a rack in a shallow roasting pan. Roast for 2 to 2½ hours. A thermometer inserted in the thickest part of the breast should register 180°F. Let stand for 20 minutes before serving.
3. Serve with turkey gravy. (Store-bought is permitted.)

## SESAME NOODLES WITH KALE
### *Serves 4 to 6*

12 ounces udon or soba noodles
1 large bunch kale, carefully
   washed and thinly sliced
2 cups broccoli florets

1 19-ounce can chickpeas, drained
2 tablespoons olive oil
2 tablespoons tamari, or to taste
2 tablespoons sesame seeds

1. Bring a large pot of water to a boil. Add the noodles and cook for 5
   minutes less than the cooking time on the package directions.
2. Add the kale, broccoli, and chickpeas to the pot, gently pressing
   them down to be fully submerged. Continue cooking, uncovered,
   for 3 to 5 minutes, until the vegetables and noodles are tender.
3. Drain the pasta and vegetables and return to the pot. Add the
   olive oil and tamari, and toss with a fork. Add the sesame seeds
   and toss again. Serve hot or at room temperature.

## CHICKEN AND ZUCCHINI SOUP
### *Serves 4 to 6*

⅓ cup uncooked brown rice
8¾ cup water, with a pinch of salt
   added
1 skinless, boneless chicken breast
   (about ¼ pound), cut into ½-
   inch pieces
2 chicken bouillon cubes
2 cups celery, sliced
2 cups leeks, well-cleaned and
   chopped, white part only

3 cloves garlic, thinly sliced
¼ cup fresh lemon juice
black pepper
2 cups zucchini, chopped into
   ½-inch pieces
2–3 tablespoons fresh cilantro or
   parsley, chopped for garnish
   (optional)

1. Put the rice into a small pan with the water. Bring to a boil,
   lower the heat, and simmer about 25 minutes, or until the water
   is absorbed. (You may add more water and continue simmering
   if the rice is not cooked enough.) Set aside.
2. In a stockpot, combine the remaining 8 cups of water, chicken,
   bouillon cubes, celery, leeks, garlic, lemon juice and pepper.
   Bring to a boil, lower the heat, and simmer for 45 minutes.

3. Add the zucchini and simmer for another 10 to 15 minutes. Add the rice and cook for a few more minutes. Adjust the seasoning. Garnish with the cilantro or parsley.

*Note:* Cilantro is preferred for this recipe, but parsley may be used. This soup will keep in the refrigerator for two to three days and may be frozen.

## GARBANZO BEAN SALAD
*Serves 4*

3 teaspoons olive oil
1 large carrot, peeled and sliced
1 stalk celery, sliced
1 medium-size red onion, thinly
    sliced
1 (15-ounce) can chickpeas,
    drained and rinsed

1 cup collard greens, shredded
1½ teaspoons ground cumin
juice of 1 lemon
sea salt
4 large romaine lettuce leaves

1. In a medium-size nonstick sauté pan, heat 1 teaspoon of the olive oil. Sauté the carrot, celery, and red onion for 4 to 6 minutes, or until soft. Mix in the chickpeas and sauté for 5 minutes.
2. Stir in the collard greens and cook until the leaves are wilted and tender. Remove from the heat. Mix in the cumin, lemon juice, remaining 2 teaspoons of olive oil, and sea salt.
3. Chill for 2 hours. To serve, spoon over lettuce leaves and serve with whole-grain bread.

## BAKED FISH À LA DEE
*Serves 4*

*This preparation is ideal for many different types of fish.*

1¾ pounds fish
¼ cup olive oil
Juice of 2 lemons
4 cloves garlic, chopped
salt and black pepper
3–4 fresh parsley sprigs, chopped
1 tablespoon dried basil

2 celery stalks, diced
2 carrots, peeled and shredded
½ yellow onion, chopped
½ cup dry white wine (you may
    add ½ cup water with wine for
    more sauce)
lemon slices, for garnish

1. Preheat the oven to 350°F.
2. Wash the fish, pat dry with a paper towel, and cut into four equal portions. Using a pastry brush, coat a shallow roasting pan or ovenproof baking dish with some of the olive oil. Place the fish in the pan and coat lightly with olive oil, using the pastry brush. Pour the lemon juice over the fish. Add salt and pepper, and set aside.
3. In a nonstick pan, heat the remaining oil. Add the parsley, garlic, and basil, and sauté for 3 to 4 minutes with the celery, carrots, and onions. Add the wine and cook for 1½ minutes (to burn off the alcohol). Remove from the heat.
4. Spoon the vegetables and liquid on top of the fish and place a slice of lemon on each portion. Place in the oven and bake for 25 minutes, or until the fish is tender.

*Note:* Add the following to make it better: *Flounder*—Sliced zucchini rounds and bread crumbs. *Sole*—Asparagus tips with chopped hard-boiled eggs. *Scrod*—Cut string beans and one slice of low-fat cheese. *Salmon\**—Fresh dill (instead of the basil); bake on a bed of fresh spinach. *Haddock*—Petite peas. *Red snapper*—Garnish with warm, bite-size, small prunes. *Mahimahi\**—Seedless grapes and sliced almonds. *Tuna\**—Bake on top of boiled sliced sweet potatoes. *Swordfish\**—Yellow squash. *Grouper*—Fresh pineapple chunks or canned pineapple chunks in their own juice.

## LEMON VINAIGRETTE

6 tablespoons fresh lemon juice
3 tablespoons safflower oil
¼ teaspoon sea salt

⅓ teaspoon black pepper
1 clove garlic, peeled and cut in half

1. Combine all of the ingredients in a covered jar, shake well, and refrigerate.
2. Remove from the refrigerator 10 to 15 minutes before using and remove the garlic. (This dressing will keep in the refrigerator for five or six days.)

*May be necessary to cook longer than the time called for in the main recipe.

## AUNT TINA'S HONEY CARROT CAKE
### Serves 12

2 cups unbleached all-purpose
flour
1 teaspoon baking powder
1 teaspoon baking soda
1 teaspoon salt
1 teaspoon ground cinnamon
1 large egg

2 large egg whites
¾ cup canola oil
1 cup honey
2½ cups carrots, grated
¼ cup raisins
¼ cup almonds, sliced and
toasted

1. Preheat the oven to 350°F. Lightly oil and flour a 9-by-13-by-2-inch pan.
2. In a large bowl, combine the flour, baking powder, baking soda, salt, and cinnamon. Set aside.
3. In another large bowl, with a wire whisk, beat the egg, egg whites, oil, and honey until well blended.
4. Stir the flour mixture into the egg mixture until well blended.
5. Using a rubber spatula, fold in the carrots and raisins. Pour into the prepared pan.
6. Bake for 50 minutes, or until a toothpick inserted into the center comes out clean. Cool on a wire rack. Remove from the pan and cut into 12 squares. Serve sprinkled with almonds.

# Several Super-Simple Sides

- Steamed string beans, topped with an olive oil-chopped garlic spread and slivered almonds.
- Baked sweet potato and squash, mashed together, with a little honey and cinnamon.
- Sautéed spinach with garlic and olive oil.
- Steamed combination of diced carrots, peas, and pearl onions.
- Low-carb pasta (such as Dreamfields) cooked as directed, with an olive oil–garlic sauce.
- Sliced cucumbers with a light cream sauce (bottled) with chives.
- Steamed broccoli florets with a lemon juice–garlic blend as a dressing.

- Brown rice or brown–wild rice blend, cooked as directed. Optional: Add steamed diced carrots and peas to the mixture, plus a pat of lightly salted butter and a teaspoon of olive oil.
- Coat steamed asparagus with a pat of butter and/or olive oil and sliced almonds.
- To a box of sugar-free Jell-O (mixed according to the package directions), add two grated carrots; allow to set.
- Raw carrot sticks, celery sticks, and olives.
- To a drained can of organic chickpeas, add diced carrots, celery, and onions.

# APPENDIX C

# Self-Hypnosis Recording for the Psoriatic

The following discourse is the basis for a self-hypnosis cassette tape that Jean Munzer, a professional hypnotist, and I developed for a few of my psoriasis patients. With specific alterations, depending on the patient, it can be adapted to meet the needs of each individual.

Most important is that the patient records the entire message *in his or her own voice,* twice on the same tape, with about a ten-second pause in between. This allows the message to enter the patient's mind just before sleep sets in and permits the patient to turn off the tape player without having to rewind. In the morning, upon awakening, he or she simply places the earphones back on, presses the Play button, and the same message is repeated. In this way, the patient receives the message at those periods when the subconscious mind is most amenable to suggestions.

*This segment of the regimen is not for everyone.* It is placed here only to give my readers and professionals an idea of the basic principles involved. Most of my patients do not need this added technique. They carry out the measures without implementing the aid of a self-hypnosis tape.

## Psoriasis Self-Hypnosis Tape Script

"I close my eyes [pause], then I take three deep breaths [pause for three deep breaths]. I will count backward from ten to one, feeling more and more relaxed with every number and every breath I take.

"Ten, nine, eight, seven, six, five, four, three, two, one.

"Following my special cleansing diet is the easiest thing in the world for me to do. I desire to eat only the foods that I know are good for me. I look upon most animal fats, sweets, hard alcohol, and the nightshades, especially tomatoes, as unhealthy to my body; therefore, I have no problem in avoiding them. It does not bother me in the least that other people can tolerate them. I know they are simply not for me. I do enjoy, however, chicken, fish, and lamb prepared any way, except fried. I avoid fried foods completely.

"When thirsty, I am quickly satisfied with a glass of pure water or seltzer, with the juice of a fresh lime or lemon, with or without ice, knowing it is very tasty and cleansing.

[For heavy smokers: "I am gradually cutting down the number of cigarettes I smoke, for I recognize tobacco as a nightshade, which, therefore, should be avoided. I am quite satisfied with just three or four cigarettes a day and see myself eliminating them altogether very soon. I find that I can feel satisfied by substituting a drink of water or seltzer for a cigarette."]

"I am enjoying my life more and more, knowing each passing day I am cleaning out unnecessary poisons and acids that my body does not need, with improved bowel and bladder evacuation.

"I know that green, leafy vegetables and fresh fruits are not only highly nutritious but aid greatly in the evacuation of the bowel and kidneys, and I enjoy eating them regularly. They help bring the body into a normal balance, filling me with more energy. As my skin clears, I focus my attention on the areas that have cleared or are clearing. If it clears in one part of my body, I know it can clear in all parts of my body. I joyfully allow my body all the time it needs and visualize myself totally clear.

"I have grown above stressful conditions by learning how to 'take things lightly.' This does not mean I minimize important matters. It means I give everything the attention it deserves, and no more. I know I can handle any situation that comes into my life, thereby making the best possible use of my energy. I am content to do what I can, then leave the rest to take care of itself. This is not only accomplishing my goals but doing it in an enjoyable, relaxed way.

"Each new day is now an adventure for me, one in which I allow only constructive, healthy thoughts to enter my consciousness. As I reflect on my former lifestyle, I recognize the changes as they occur in my life in the form of revitalized health, renewed ambition, and restored energy.

"Every time I hear this recorded message, it is deeply engraved into my subconscious and consequently manifests in my everyday life.

"I will now count forward from one to ten. At the count of ten, I will open my eyes, feeling well rested, and turn off the recorder. I have renewed motivation to achieve my goal of freeing myself of psoriasis every time I listen to this personal message.

"One, two, three, four, five, six, seven, eight, nine, ten."

*Author's note:* Henry Leo Bolduc is author of the book *Self-Hypnosis: Creating Your Own Destiny*. It may be obtained by writing to the ARE Bookstore, Virginia Beach, VA 23451, (757) 428-3588 ext. 7231

# APPENDIX D

# Product Suppliers

The following suppliers have available the most important items required in cases of psoriasis, psoriatic arthritis, and eczema. They include the following: slippery elm bark powder, American yellow saffron tea, Glyco-Thymoline, Atomodine, Dead Sea salts, the tri-salts (sulphur, cream of tartar, Rochelle salts—trade name Sulflax), Almond Glow or Aura Glow (both olive oil–peanut oil mixtures), and castor oil.

**Baar Products**
P.O. Box 60
Dowingtown, PA 19335
Tel: 610-873-4591
Toll-Free: 800-269-2502
Fax: 610-873-7945
www.baar.com
Catalog available on request.

**The Heritage Store**
314 Laskin Road
P.O. Box 444
Virginia Beach, VA 23458
Tel: 757-428-0100
Toll-Free: 800-862-2923
www.caycecures.com
Catalog available on request.

Most other items such as hydrophilic ointment, Epsom salts, witch hazel, Vaseline, and similar products can be obtained or ordered from local pharmacies.

# ACKNOWLEDGMENTS

This volume was made possible by the kind and generous assistance of the following individuals and organizations to help me turn this dream into a reality: Dada J. P. Vaswani, Elsa Reinhardt, Johanna Reinhardt Bayati, Marie Diehl, JoAnne MacBeth, Annette Shandolow-Hassell, Sunil and Beena Ahuja (At Last Sportswear, Inc.), Justine Skiba, Ingrid and Klaus A. Werner, Leslie Del Rosso, Reva and Stanley I. Elkins, Elisabeth and Peter Henderson, Sharon Solomon, Joanne Richmond, Sydney and Stephen Salmieri, Jonas Honig, Norbert Mester, Jeanette Thomas Mundt, Jim Windsor, and all of my friends at the Association for Research and Enlightenment and the Edgar Cayce Foundation, Virginia Beach, Virginia.

I would also like to thank the patients themselves for their cooperation in allowing me to document and publish their personal case histories and photographs.

Finally, thanks to Marjorie May for creating menus for the seven-day sample menus.

## In Memoriam

My dear mother and father, Nettie and John J. Pagano, Esq.; Hugh Lynn Cayce; Gladys Davis Turner; Gina Cerminara; Tony Merola; Al Riecker; H. J. Reilly; Thea Wheelwright; Martha and Nick Nicklin; Alice and Judge Harold Gilmore; and my beloved Shane.

# NOTES

## 1. Psoriasis: The "Inside" Story

3  *"There is a cure"*  Edgar Cayce Reference #2455-2 (Virginia Beach: The Edgar Cayce Foundation, 1971).

5  *It is within*  Ibid., #3373-1.

6  *The Leaky Gut Syndrome*  Zolton Rona, "Leaky Gut or Permeable Bowel Syndrome," Life Enthusiast Co-op, www.life-enthusiast.com/index/Articles/Rona, accessed May 21, 2008.

9  *improper coordination in*  Frederick D. Lansford, "Commentary on Psoriasis," in *Physician's Reference Notebook,* ed. William A. McGarey (Virginia Beach: ARE Press, 1968), 189—extracted from References #5016-1 and #622-1.

9  *Doubtless, some of the conditions*  Israel S. Kleiner, *Human Biochemistry,* 4th ed. (St. Louis, MO: C. V. Mosby Co., 1954), 543.

## 3. About Psoriasis

20  *"Scientists do not yet"*  U.S. Department of Health, Education and Welfare, National Institutes of Health, *Psoriasis,* DHEW Publication No. NIH 77-1104 (Washington, DC: U.S. Government Printing Office, 1977).

20  *perspiratory system*  Edgar Cayce Reference #3373-1 (Virginia Beach: The Edgar Cayce Foundation, 1971).

23  *Exfoliative psoriasis usually*  John Franklin, "Scaly Eruptions," in *French's Index of Differential Diagnosis,* 7th ed., ed. Arthur H. Douthwaite (Baltimore, MD: Williams and Wilkins, 1954), 732.

23  *"Most surveys indicate"*  Ronald Marks, *Psoriasis: A Guide to One of the Commonest Skin Diseases* (New York: Arco Publishing, 1981), 32.

24  *In Sweden, however*  L. Hellgren, "Statistical, Clinical and Laboratory Investigation of 255 Psoriatics and Matched Healthy Controls," in *Psoriasis* (Stockholm: Acta Dermatovener 44, 1964), 191–207.

24  *Dr. Litt classifies psoriasis*  John O'Rourke, "Vitamin A vs. Psoriasis," *Let's Live* (April 1983), 24.

24    *there is an associated family*    George M. Lewis, *Practical Dermatology for Medical Students and General Practitioners* (Philadelphia: W. B. Saunders Co., 1952), 80.

24    *It is common in East African*    A. R. H. B. Verhagen and J. W. Koten, "Psoriasis in Kenya," *Archives of Dermatology* 96 39–41 (1967).

30    *"although cyclosporine is"*    Nicholas J. Lowe, "Systemic Treatment of Severe Psoriasis—the Role of Cyclosporine," *New England Journal of Medicine* 324, no. 5 (Jan. 31, 1991): 333–334.

## 5. Internal Cleansing

36    *Chronic constipation and*    Frederick D. Lansford Jr., "Commentary on Psoriasis," in *Physician's Reference Notebook*, ed. William A. McGarey (Virginia Beach: The ARE Press, 1968), 189.

36    *"When the contents of"*    Francis M. Pottenger, *Symptoms of Visceral Disease,* 7th ed. (St. Louis, MO: C. V. Mosey Co., 1953), 272.

46    *The liver and the kidneys*    Henry G. Bieler, *Food Is Your Best Medicine* (New York: Random House, 1973), 42–43.

47    *"in all cases of toxemia"*    Pottenger, *Symptoms,* p. 280.

58    *"Vitamin B, and other"*    Charles Best and Norman Taylor, *The Living Body: A Text in Human Physiology*, 3rd ed. (New York: Henry Holt and Co., 1952), 381.

62    *Fiber-rich foods bind water*    Jeffrey Bland, *Intestinal Toxicity and Inner Cleansing* (New Canaan, CT: Keats Publishing), 15–18, 20–21.

## 6. Diet and Nutrition Basics

71    *nature demands that*    Edgar Cayce Reference #306-3 (Virginia Beach: The Edgar Cayce Foundation, 1971).

71    *A person's blood should*    Israel S. Kleiner, *Human Biochemistry*, 4th ed. (St. Louis, MO: C. V. Mosby Co., 1954), 543.

77    *When toxemia is*    Francis M. Pottenger, *Symptoms of Visceral Disease,* 7th ed. (St. Louis, MO: C. V. Mosby Co., 1953), 144.

78    *"eczema-like skin condition"*    Adelle Davis, *Let's Get Well* (New York: Harcourt, Brace and World, 1965), 156.

80    *presents these charts*    Michel Gauguelin, *How Atmospheric Conditions Affect Your Health* (New York: Stein and Day, 1971.)

84    *in some cases of psoriasis*    Eugene J. Van Scott and Eugene M. Farber, *Dermatology in General Medicine* (New York: McGraw-Hill, 1971), 226.

87    *there is no indication*    "More Than One Way to Skin a Chicken," *Tufts University Diet and Nutrition Letter* 8, no. 10 (1990): 7.

104    *six out of six patients*    Melvyn R. Werbach, *Nutritional Influence on Illness* (New Canaan, CT: Keats Publishing, 1988), 372.

107    *Food items to consume*    *Tufts University Diet and Nutrition Letter,* March 1997.

## 7. Herbal Teas

113 *Place about a quarter* Readers who wish a more detailed account of the benefits of saffron tea are advised to purchase *An Edgar Cayce Health Anthology*, which includes a comprehensive article, "The Healing Powers of Saffron Tea," by Robert O. Clapp, and may be ordered from the ARE Bookstore, Box 595, Virginia Beach, VA 23451; phone: 1-757-428-3588.

115 *The Chinese have long* Richard Lucas, *Secrets of the Chinese Herbalists* (West Nyack, NY: Parker Publishing Co., 1977), 191–92.

117 *Numerous benefits have been* Jethro Kloss, *Back to Eden: A Human Interest Story of Health and Restoration to Be Found in Herb, Root, and Bark* (New York: Beneficial Books, 1971), 212–13.

## 8. The Role of the Spine

119 *"Diseases cannot be divided"* Francis M. Pottenger, *Symptoms of Visceral Disease,* 7th ed. (St. Louis, MO: C. V. Mosby Co., 1953), 9.

124 *"The structures of the skin"* Ibid., p. 410.

126 *practical results* J. E. Bourdillon, *Spinal Manipulation*, 3rd ed. (London: William Heinemann Medical Books Ltd., 1982), 2.

## 10. Right Thinking: The Role of the Mind

145 *"Of all the beautiful"* James Allen, *As a Man Thinketh* (Mt. Vernon, NY: Peter Pauper Press), 9.

146 *Everything begins with an* emotion Thomas Troward, *The Edinburgh Lectures on Mental Science* (New York: Dodd, Mead and Company, 1909), 85.

148 *"is to keep the imagination"* Ibid., p. 84.

154 *"Every day in"* Émile Coué, *Self-Mastery through Conscious Autosuggestion* (London: WCIA, Unwin Hyman, 1921).

155 *"But people say"* Thomas Troward, *The Hidden Power and Other Papers upon Mental Science* (New York: R. M. McBride and Co., 1921), 97–98.

## 11. The Emotional Factor

163 *"The Negative Emotion"* Manly P. Hall, *Healing, the Divine Art* (Los Angeles: Philosophical Research Society, 1943), 260, 261.

164 *"The causes of skin disorders"* Ted A. Grossbart, "Bringing Peace to Embattled Skin," *Psychology Today,* February 1982, p. 55. Ted A. Grossbart, PhD, has also coauthored the book *Skin Deep: A Mind/Body Program for Healthy Skin* with Carl Sherman, PhD (New York: William Morrow, 1986).

165 *"The skin lives"* Ibid., p. 59.

168 *"Such emotions as fear"* Francis M. Pottenger, *Symptoms of Visceral Disease,* 7th ed. (St. Louis, MO: C. V. Mosby Co., 1953), 135.

169 *"Harmony in the mind"* Hall, *Healing,* p. 238.

169   *"Anger causes poisons"*   Edgar Cayce Reference #281–54 (Virginia Beach: The Edgar Cayce Foundation, 1971).
170   *"those who attend"*   *Time*, June 24, 1996, p. 60.
171   *"Influences from within"*   Edgar Cayce, *A Search for God,* compiled by the Study Groups of the Association for Research and Enlightenment (Virginia Beach, 1942–1950), 76.

## 16. The Arthritic Connection: Psoriatic Arthritis

230   *Atomodine was rarely*   Members of the ARE can obtain more precise details on Atomodine by consulting the appropriate Circulating File. The ARE publication *An Edgar Cayce Home Medicine Guide,* available to the general public, contains a very informative article on Atomodine (ARE Bookstore, Box 595, Virginia Beach, VA 23451).

## 18. What about the Failures?

252   *"My health!"*   Wyn Wachhorst, *Thomas Alva Edison—An American Myth* (Cambridge, MA: MIT Press, 1981), 164.

# BIBLIOGRAPHY

Allen, James. *As a Man Thinketh*. Kansas City, MO: Andrew McMeel Pub., 1999.

Bach, Marcus. *The Chiropractic Story*. Los Angeles, CA: De Vorss and Co., 1968.

Best, Charles, and Norman Taylor. *The Living Body,* 3rd ed. New York: Henry Holt and Co., 1952.

————. *The Physiological Basis of Medical Practice,* 6th ed. Baltimore, MD: The Williams and Wilkins Company, 1955.

Bieler, Henry G. *Food Is Your Best Medicine*. New York: Random House, 1973.

Bland, Jeffrey. *Intestinal Toxicity and Inner Cleansing*. New Canaan, CT: Keats Publishing, 1987.

Bloom, William, and Don W. Fawcett. *A Textbook of Histology,* 10th ed. Philadelphia: W. B. Saunders Company, 1975.

Bolduc, Henry Leo. *Self-Hypnosis: Creating Your Own Destiny*. Virginia Beach: ARE Press, 1985, by the Edgar Cayce Foundation.

Bolton, Brett. *An Edgar Cayce Encyclopedia of Foods for Health and Healing*. Virginia Beach: ARE Press, 1997.

Bourdillon, J. E. *Spinal Manipulation,* 3rd ed. New York: Appleton-Century Crofts, 1982.

Brody, Jane E. "Emotions Found to Influence Nearly Every Human Ailment." *New York Times,* May 24, 1983.

Cayce, Edgar. *Readings*. Virginia Beach: The Edgar Cayce Foundation, 1971, Reference 2455-2, Reference 2002-1, Reference 306-3, Reference 281-54.

Childers, Norman F. *Arthritis—Childers' Diet to Stop It*. Gainesville, FL: Horticultural Publications, 1977.

*Circulating Files on Psoriasis*. Virginia Beach: ARE Press, 1971, by the Edgar Cayce Foundation, vols. 1, 2.

Coué, Émile. *Self-Mastery through Conscious Autosuggestion*. London: G. Allen & Unwin, 1984.

Davis, Adelle. *Let's Get Well*. New York: Harcourt, Brace and World, 1965.

Douthwaite, Arthur H., ed. *French's Index of Differential Diagnosis*, 7th ed. Bristol, Eng.: John Wright and Sons, Ltd., 1954.

Gauguelin, Michael. *How Atmospheric Conditions Affect Your Health*. New York: Stein and Day Publishers, 1971.

Gray, Henry. *Gray's Anatomy*, 26th ed. Edited by Charles Mayo Goss. Philadelphia: Lea & Febiger, 1954.

Grossbart, Ted A. "Bringing Peace to Embattled Skin," *Psychology Today,* February 1982.

Hall, Manly P. *Healing, the Divine Art*. Los Angeles: Philosophical Research Society, Inc., 1943.

*Healing Power of Vitamins, Minerals and Herbs, The*. Pleasantville, NY: The Reader's Digest Association, 1999.

Hellgren, L. "Statistical, Clinical and Laboratory Investigation of 255 Psoriatics and Matched Healthy Controls," in *Psoriasis*. Stockholm: Acta Dermatovener 44, 1964.

Houssay, Bernard A. *Human Physiology*, 2nd ed. New York: McGraw-Hill Book Company, 1955.

Jensen, Bernard, and Sylvia Bell. *Tissue Cleansing through Bowel Management*, 6th ed. Escondido, CA: Bernard Jensen, DC, 1981.

Kleiner, Israel S. *Human Biochemistry,* 4th ed. St. Louis, MO: C. V. Mosby Co., 1954.

Kloss, Jethro. *Back to Eden*. New York: Laurer Books, 1971.

Lansford, Frederick D. "Commentary on Psoriasis" in *Physician's Reference Notebook*, ed. by William A. McGarey. Virginia Beach: ARE Press, 1968.

Lewis, George M. *Practical Dermatology*. Philadelphia: W. B. Saunders Company, 1952.

Lowe, Nicholas J. "Systemic Treatment of Severe Psoriasis—the Role of Cyclosporine," *New England Journal of Medicine,* 324, no. 5 January 31, 1991.

Lucas, Richard. *Secrets of the Chinese Herbalists*. West Nyack, NY: Parker Publishing Co., 1977.

Marks, Ronald, *Psoriasis*. New York: Arco Publishing, 1981.

Maximow, Alexander A., and William Bloom. *A Textbook of Histology,* 6th ed. Philadelphia and London: W. B. Saunders Company, 1952.

McGarey, William A. "Indigestion." *Health Care Report* 1, no. 4. Virginia Beach: Edgar Cayce Foundation.

———. "Olive Oil May Protect the Heart." *Pathways to Health*. Medical Research Bulletin 7, no. 3. Phoenix, AZ: ARE Clinic, Inc.

———. "Rheumatoid Arthritis." *Pathways to Health*. Medical Research Bulletin 1, no. 2. June/July 1979. Phoenix, AZ: ARE Clinic, Inc.

Monroe, Anne Shannon. *Singing in the Rain*. Garden City, NY: Sun Dial Press, 1926.

"More than One Way to Skin a Chicken." *Tufts University Diet and Nutrition Letter.* Food for Thought 8, no. 10, December 1990.

O'Rourke, John. "Vitamin A vs. Psoriasis." *Let's Live,* April 1983.

*Pathogenesis of Visceral Disease Following Vertebral Lesions*. Chicago, IL: American Osteopathic Association, 1948.

"Pathways to Health," *Medical Research Bulletin* 1, no. 2, June/July 1979. Phoenix, AZ: ARE Clinic.

Pottenger, Francis M., *Symptoms of Visceral Disease*, 7th ed. St. Louis, MO: C. V. Mosby Co., 1953.

*Psoriasis*, DHEW Publication No. NIH, 77-1104. Washington, DC: U.S. Government Printing Office, 1977.

Reilly, Harold J., and Ruth Hagy Brod. *The Edgar Cayce Handbook for Health through Drugless Therapy*. New York: Macmillan Publishing Co., 1975.

Scott, Eugene J., and Eugene M. Farber. *Dermatology in General Medicine*. New York: McGraw-Hill, 1971.

"Shucking the Myth about Cholesterol in Shellfish." *Tufts University Diet and Nutrition Letter*. Food for Thought 5, no. 4, June 1987.

Sugrue, Thomas. *There Is a River*, rev. ed. New York: Holt, Rinehart and Winston Publishers, 1945.

Troward, Thomas. *The Edinburgh Lectures on Mental Science*. New York: Dodd, Mead and Company, 1909.

———. *The Hidden Power*. New York: Dodd, Mead and Company, 1921.

Verhagen, A. R. H. B., and J. W. Koten. "Psoriasis in Kenya." *Archives of Dermatology* 9639-41. Chicago: 1967.

Wachhorst, Wyn. *Thomas Alva Edison—an American Myth*. Cambridge, MA: MIT Press, 1981.

Werbach, Melvyn R. *Nutritional Influence on Illness*. New Canaan, CT: Keats Publishing, 1988.

Wolberg, Lewis. *Medical Hypnosis*. New York: Grune and Stratton, 1948.

Zinsser, William. *On Writing Well*. New York: Harper and Row, 1976.

# ILLUSTRATION CREDITS

All images are from the author's personal collection except the following:

Figures 3-1, 5-1, 5-3, 8-4: *Gray's Anatomy* 26th edition, Lea & Febiger Publishers, Philadelphia, PA, 1954—reprinted by permission; 30th edition, edited by Carmine D. Clemente, 1985.

Figure 3-2: *Dermatology in General Medicine* by Fitzpatrick et al., New York, NY: McGraw-Hill Book Company, 1971, p. 221. Reproduced by permission.

Figures 5-2A, 5-2B, and 5-2C: *Tissue Cleansing through Bowel Management* by Dr. Bernard Jensen, DC, PhD, and Sylvia Bell, copyright 1981, 6th edition. Published by Bernard Jensen, DC, Route 1, Box 52, Escondido, CA 92025. Reproduced by permission.

Figures 8-1, 8-2: Chiropractic Public Relations (CPR), 141 Blauvelt Street, Teaneck, NJ 07666. Reprinted by permission.

# INDEX

Page numbers in *italics* refer to illustrations.

acanthosis, 19
acid-alkaline balance, 41–42, 71
  above-/below-ground vegetables
    and, 275–276
  alkaline vs. acid formers, 73–76
  arthritis and, 224–226, 231
  80/20 percent food ratio and,
    71–72, 100–101, 272–274
  food combinations to avoid, 280
  toxemia and, 77
activated vitamin D cream, 28–29
adjustment. *See* spinal adjustment
age factors, 23
alcohol, 7, 99, 227, 253–254
alkaline foods. *See* acid-alkaline
    balance
Allen, James, 145
allergies, 102–103, 117, 130, 217–219
almonds, 61
alpha-lipoic acid, 105
alpha visualization, 155–156
"AMA Cautions against Tanning"
    (AP), 136
American Medical Association
    (AMA), 86, 93, 136
American yellow saffron tea, 7–8, 97,
    111, 112–113, 264
  for eczema, 239

preparation of, 113–115
saffron water, 63, 113
steam treatments with, 63–64,
    114, 217
*Anatomy of an Illness* (Cousins), 12
anger, 229
antacids, 219
antibiotics, 6
antiperspirant, 178–179
apple cider vinegar
  in diet, 84
  as external application, 135, 137
  as hair rinse, 175
  for itchy scalp, 174
apples, 218
  acid-alkaline balance and, 74
  Apple and Butternut Squash
    Soup, 297
  as laxative, 58
  Three-Day Apple Diet, 53–56,
    102–103, 263
apricots, 58
Aquaphore, 187
*Archives of Dermatology*, 112
*ARE Journal*, 258
aromatic retinoid, 28
arteriosclerosis, 78
arthritis, 40–41

arthritis (*continued*)
 dairy and, 88–89
 diet and, 56
 generalized/erythrodermic psoriasis
  and, 22
 nightshades and, 81
 types of, 223
 *See also* psoriatic arthritis
arthritis mutilans, 223
articular facets, 121
artificial sweeteners, 93
*As a Man Thinketh* (Allen), 145
ascending colon, 37, 52
Associated Press (AP), 61, 136, 225
Association for Research and
  Enlightenment (ARE),
  11, 228, 258
asteatotic dermatitis ("winter itch"),
  228–229
asymmetric oligoarthritis, 223
atmospheric conditions. *See* humidity
Atomodine, 230, 231
*Atropa belladonna,* 80–81
attitude, 3, 7, 268–271
 emotions and, 160–171
 right thinking and, 145–159
 success of treatment and, 254–256
 toxins and, 48–49
Aunt Tina's Honey Carrot Cake, 301
Auspitz sign, 20
autoimmune disease, 5. *See also* leaky
  gut syndrome
Aveeno bath, 137
avocados, 74

Baar Products, 8, 177
bacon, 88
Bag Balm, 187
Baked Fish à la Dee, 299–300
Baker's P&S Liquid, 133, 174
baking soda. *See* sodium bicarbonate
  (baking soda)
ballooned sigmoid colon, 38

bananas, 56, 74, 227
Barbara's Broccoli Dip, 295
base. *See* acid-alkaline balance
beliefs, 148–150, 170. *See also*
  right thinking
belladonna, 81
Best, Charles, 58
beverages, 94–99, 280–281. *See also*
  teas; water intake
Bieler, Henry G., 4, 46
birth-control pills, 7
black tea, 98
blood
 acid-alkaline balance and, 71–72
 kidneys and, 41–42
 purifying, 36
 wine and, 99
Bourdillon, J. E., 126
bowels. *See* internal cleansing
breakfast, 277–279, 283–288
breathing exercises, 43, 49, 64–65
"Bringing Peace to Embattled Skin"
  (Grossbart), 164–165
broccoli
 about, 218
 Barbara's Broccoli Dip, 295
Brocq, Louis, 161
Brody, Jane E., 161–162
Broiled Flounder Fillets, 296
Broiled Lamb Patties with
  Marinade, 291
Brown Rice with Lentils, 294–295

calamari, 84
calcium, 89
Canadian National Consumer
  Institute, 108
carbohydrates, 7
Carbolated Vaseline, 178
carbonated drinks, 98–99
carbon dioxide, 43
carob, 92–93
Carr, William Kearny, 256

carrots
    about, 218, 224
    Aunt Tina's Honey Carrot
        Cake, 301
    Roasted Carrots and Parsnips,
        293–294
castor oil
    for external application, 114, 132
    Fletcher's Castoria, 58–59, 243
    packs, 45
cathartics. *See* internal cleansing;
    laxatives
Cayce, Edgar, 3, 32–33, 271
    on arthritis, 224–226
    Association for Research and
        Enlightenment (ARE), 11,
        228, 258
    on Atomodine, 230
    on cause of psoriasis, 6, 9
    on curing psoriasis, 71
    on diet, 82, 99, 108
    on eczema, 238, 239, 249
    Edgar Cayce Foundation, 9, 11, 226
    on emotions, 160, 168–169
    on Glyco-Thymoline, 138
    on religious beliefs, 171
    on source of psoriasis, 4
    on spine, 119
    on steam baths, 62
    on tri-salts, 60
    on visualization, 149
Cayce/Pagano Regimen, 30–31,
        32–35
    future of psoriasis treatment and,
        267–271
    goals for, 262–266
    recurrence of psoriasis and,
        257–261
    response to, 1–2, 11–16, 32–33,
        144, 194–195, 215–221,
        250–256
    *See also* diet; external applications;
        internal cleansing

celery, 224
celiac disease, 90
Center for Science in the Public
        Interest, 92–93
cereals, 90, 278
cervical curve, 121
chamomile tea, 98, 112, 117
Charlton Tuna Salad, 290–291
chicken, 87–88
    Chicken and Zucchini Soup,
        298–299
    Oriental Chicken Salad, 292–293
Childers, Norman F., 81, 82, 226
children
    eczema in, 243–246
    psoriasis in teenagers, 259–261
chiropractic, 123, 125–128
    for eczema, 239
    for "poker spine," 233–234
    *See also* spine
cholesterol
    high-fiber foods and, 61
    lecithin and, 78
    olive oil and, 60
chyme, 8
cirrhosis of the liver, 98
citrus fruits/juices, 278, 280
    acid-alkaline balance and, 73, 74
    Citrus Diet, 54, 55
    in combination with grains, 91
    orange juice "sandwich," 59
clothing
    eczema and, 242–243
    for hands/feet, 182–183, 191, 232
    pajama shower/bath, 220–221
    synthetic fabrics as, 143
cloth wraps, for external
        applications, 131
coccyx, 121–123, *122*
cod liver oil, 236–237
coffee, 7, 95–97, 278
Cold Tuna-Noodle Salad, 296
Coleslaw, 294

colon, *8*
  anatomy, *37, 37–41, 38, 39, 40,* 52
  colitis, *39*
  colonic irrigation, 50–52, 263
  *See also* internal cleansing
common vulgaris (plaque-type)
    psoriasis, 21, 22, 206–207
*Concurrence, The* (Carr), 256
conscious mind, 152–155
constipation. *See* elimination
contact sports, 64
copper, 105
Cornell University, 82
cosmetic tanning, 136
cotton clothing, 143, 242–243
cotton gloves, 183
Coué, Émile, 152–155, 155
Cousins, Norman, 12
Culmone, Minnie, 12
Culmone, William, 12–13, 133,
  258–259
"cure," for psoriasis, 268–271
Cuticura
  ointment, 133, 134, 216
  shampoo treatment, 133, 175, 177
  soap, 114, 133
cyclosporine, 29–30
cytotoxic test, 103

dairy, 88–89, 98, 278
  eczema and, 241
  salt in, 225–226
Dalai Lama, 171
Davis, Adelle, 78
"Deadly Seven," 109
Dead Sea
  benefits of, 29
  salts baths, 134
degenerative joint disease (DJD), 223
dehydration, 219–221
Deluxe Acorn Squash, 291
deodorant, 178–179
depression, 7

derma/dermis, 18–19, *19*
descending colon, *37,* 52
detoxification, 32–33, 49–50, 65–66
dialysis of the blood, 28, 42
"die-off" period, 219
diet, 48, 67–71, 107–110, 263
  acid-alkaline balance in, 41–42,
    71–77, 80, 100–101, 224–226,
    231, 272–276, 280
  adhering to, 100, 101, 105–106,
    253–254
  beverages in, 94–99, 280–281
    (*See also* water intake)
  dining out and, 106–107
  fiber in, 60–62
  food allergies and, 102–103, 117,
    130, 217–219
  foods/food combinations to avoid,
    274–275, 280–281
  meal planning principles, 277–279
  nightshades in, 7, 68–69, 75,
    80–82, 226
  parasites in, 7
  portion size, 101, 102, 215
  proteins and starches, 276–277
  recipes, 289–302
  salad dressings and olive oil in,
    83–84
  sample menus, 283–288
  supplements in, 103–105 (*See also*
    minerals; vitamins)
  Three-Day Apple Diet, 53–56,
    102–103, 263
  weight loss and, 100–101, 215
  *See also* teas; *individual names of*
    *foods; individual names of nutrients*
Diffey, Brian, 29
digestive tract anatomy, 4–9, *5, 8.*
  *See also* intestinal tract
dinner, 279, 283–288
dish washing, 182–183
distilled water, 57
diverticula, *39*

diverticulosis, 90
dogs, 65
dressings
   in diet, 83–84
   Lemon Vinaigrette, 300
*Dr. John's Healing Psoriasis
      Cookbook . . . Plus!* (Pagano), 93,
      101, 190, 282
dual therapy, 27
duodenal-jejenal junction (flexure), 123
duodenum, 4, *5, 8*
dye, for hair, 172

eczema, 18, 40–41, 238
   acid-alkaline balance and, 72
   alcohol and, 99
   case studies, 238–243, 244–246
   diet and, 56, 105
   of genital area, 138
   psoriasis correlation, 246–249
   teas for, 112
   in young children, 243–246
Eddy, David M., 16
Edgar Cayce Foundation, 9, 11, 226
*Edinburgh Lectures on Mental Science*
      (Troward), 146–147
Edison, Thomas A., 252
eggplant, 81, 82
eggs, 278
80/20 percent food ratio, 71–72,
      100–101, 272–274
electrical stimulation
   of spine, 128
   as topical therapy, 138–139, 142,
      234, 235
electric hair dryers, 175
electric heat caps, 172–178
electric heating pads, 232–233
elimination
   constipation, 7, 36
   eczema and, 241
   enemas and, 50–53, 60, 143, 219,
      227, 263

olive oil–tincture of myrrh massage
      and, 139–140
   toilet habits, 37–41, 47–48
   *See also* internal cleansing; laxatives
Ellis, Charles, 29–30
emotions
   awareness of, 164–165, 168–169
   influence on health, 160–164
   multi-disciplinary approaches to,
      169–170
   positive approach to, 171
   religious beliefs and, 170–171
   self-image and, 169–170
   self-sabotage and, 165–166
   stress and, 166–167, 229
"Emotions Found to Influence Nearly
      Every Human Ailment" (Brody),
      161–162
emulsions. *See* external applications
enemas, 219, 263
   for arthritis, 227
   high colonic irrigation and,
      50–52, 227
   home use of, 52–53, 143
   olive oil as, 60
Eno Salts, 59
enzymes, 7, 108
epidermis, 18–19, *19, 20, 32–33*
Epsom salts bath, 63, 134, 216,
      263–264
   for arthritis, 232
   drying effect of, 228
   for hands/feet, 181–182
esophagus, 4, *5*
essential fatty acids, 105
exercise
   for arthritis, 235
   internal cleansing and, 64–65
   for lungs, 43–44
exfoliative psoriasis, 21, 23
expectancy, 158–159
external applications, 27, 129–130,
      141–143

external applications (*continued*)
  Aveeno bath, 137
  Baker's P&S Liquid, 133, 174
  castor oil, 45, 114, 132
  Cuticura products, 114, 133, 134,
    175, 177, 216
  Dead Sea salts bath, 134
  for eczema, 243
  electrical stimulation as, 138–139,
    234, 235
  Epsom salts bath, 63, 134,
    181–182, 216, 228, 263–264
  fume/steam baths, 62–64, 135,
    137–138, 142
  Glyco-Thymoline, 60, 135,
    137–138, 174, 176, 217
  for hands/feet, 180–191
  during healing period, 220–221
  hydrophilic ointment, 140–141
  Listerine, 137–138, 174, 175, 176
  natural sunlight, 135–136
  olive oil mixtures, 130–132,
    139–140
  Ray's Ointment, 133, 174, 178,
    239, 242
  Resinol, 132, 133
  sodium bicarbonate (baking soda),
    132, 137
  synthetic fabrics and, 143,
    242–243 (*See also* clothing)
  ultrasound, 138–139
  ultraviolet light, 28, 51, 129,
    135–136, 142, 268
  Vaseline, 132, 133
  vitamin E, 133–134
  witch hazel, 62, 64, 137–138

face, psoriasis on, 178–179
family, as support system, 216, 251
fear, 163
feet
  psoriasis on, 180–182, 183–190
  psoriasis under nails, 190–191

figs, 58–59
First International Conference on
    Holistic Health and Medicine, 25
fish, 86–88, 107
  Baked Fish à la Dee, 299–300
  Broiled Flounder Fillets, 296
  Charlton Tuna Salad, 290–291
  Cold Tuna-Noodle Salad, 296
  oils, 108–109, 236–237
  Poached Orange Roughy with
    Spinach, 293
  shellfish, 84–86, 185
flaxseed oil, 108–109
Fletcher's Castoria, 58–59, 243
flexural psoriasis, 21, 22
Flounder Fillets, Broiled, 296
*Food Is Your Best Medicine* (Bieler), 46
fowl, 86–88
free radicals, 84
Fresh Fruit Diet, 54, 55–56
fruits, 107
  acid-alkaline balance and, 73–76
  citrus, 54, 55, 73, 74, 91, 278, 280
  flour and, 280
  fruit juices, 95
  as laxatives, 58
  to replace sweets, 92–93
  *See also* diet
fume baths, 62–63, 135, 137–138
fungal mycotoxins, 7

Galland, Leo, 236
Garbanzo Bean Salad, 299
generalized/erythrodermic psoriasis,
    21, 22, 202–203, 208–209,
    212–214
genital area, 138, 217
Genova Diagnostics, 10
germinative cell population, 19–20, *20*
Gillette wraparound heat unit,
    232–233
"Glorious Seven," 109–110
gloves, 182–183

glutamine supplement, 236
gluten, 90
"glut" response, 48
glycoalkaloids, 82
Glyco-Thymoline
    external use, 60, 135, 137–138,
        174, 176, 217
    internal use, 75, 77, 231
glycyrrhetinic acid cream, 105
goat's milk, 241
Goeckerman regimen, 27, 268
gout, 84
grains, 89–92
Grape Diet, 54, 55
grape seed extract, 105
Green Goddess Soup, 292
green tea, 98, 108
Green Vegetable Casserole,
    295–296
Grossbart, Ted A., 164–165
Grundy, Scott, 84
"guardian at the gate" principle, 150
guttate psoriasis, 21, 22, 210–211

hair. See scalp
Hall, Manly Palmer, 157, 163,
    168–169
hands
    psoriasis of, 180–193
    psoriasis under nails, 190–191
    ultrasound for, 139
hate, 163
Healing, the Divine Art (Hall), 163
Healing Power of Vitamins, Minerals,
    and Herbs, The (Reader's Digest),
    104–105
healing process
    allowing time for, 144, 194–195,
        215–221
    case studies of, 195–200, 201,
        202–203, 204–205, 206–207,
        208–209, 210–211, 212–214
    failure to respond to, 250–256

future of psoriasis treatment and,
    267–271
    goals for, 262–266
    recurrence and, 257–261
heat caps/mitts/boots, 142
heating pads, 232–233
heat prostration, 63
hemodialysis, 28
hepatic cells, 36, 44
herbal teas. See teas
hereditary factors, 7
Heritage Store, 8
Herxheimer reaction, 34–35,
    219–221
Hidden Power, The (Troward), 155
high colonic irrigation, 50–52, 227
high-fiber foods, 60–62, 90.
    See also diet
Hippocrates, 110, 128
Hoke, Margaret, 87
Holick, Michael, 28–29
holism
    external applications and, 142
    holistic healing, 33–34
    "oneness" concept of, 119–120
homeostasis, 33
honey, 92
hot bed sheet applications, 220
How Atmospheric Conditions Affect Your
    Health (Tromp), 80
humidity
    acid-alkaline balance and, 80
    humidifiers for home use, 142
    "winter itch" and, 228
hunger, 215
Hutner, S. H., 98
hydrophilic ointment, 140–141
hydrotherapy, defined, 235
hyperkeratosis, 190–191
hypnosis, 153–155

Ikemi, Y., 169
ileitis, 116–117

ileocecal valve, 8
ileum, 5, 5, 8–9
imagination, will and, 148–150, 155
imaging, 156–157
incontinence, urinary, 42
India, 25
Innerclean, 59
innervation, of skin, 124
internal cleansing, 36
  colon anatomy, 37, 37–41,
    38, 39, 40
  detoxification and, 49–50,
    65–66
  enemas, 50–52, 52–53, 60, 143,
    219, 227, 263
  exercise and, 64–65
  fume/steam baths for, 62–64
  high colonic irrigation,
    50–52, 227
  kidney anatomy, 41–42,
    46–47
  liver anatomy, 44–45, 45, 46–47
  natural cathartics/laxatives,
    49, 57–62, 79, 242
  skin and lung anatomy, 42–44,
    46–47
  Three-Day Apple Diet for, 53–56,
    102–103, 263
  toxic buildup and, 47–49
  water intake and, 56–57
intestinal tract, 4
  eczema and, 238
  ileitis, 116–117
  intestinal permeability (leaky gut
    syndrome), 2, 5, 6–10, 115–117,
    120, 236
  spine and, 120
intravenous feeding, 68–69, 219
iodine, 230
itching, 18, 137
  Glyco-Thymoline for, 231
  during healing process, 217
  itchy scalp, 174

"winter itch," 228–229
  See also external applications
Jacquet, Leonard, 161
jejunum, 5, 5, 8
jelly, 278
Jensen, Bernard, 37
Jerusalem artichokes, 227
Johns Hopkins Medical School, 95
joints, swelling of, 231–233. See also
  arthritis; psoriatic arthritis
Journal of the American Medical
  Association, 93
juice, 278
  home preparation of, 143
  vitamin assimilation and, 74
  See also diet; fruits; vegetables

ketchup, 196
kidneys, 41–42, 46–47
Koebner phenomenon, 26
kyphotic curve, 121

lamb
  about, 86–88
  Broiled Lamb Patties with
    Marinade, 291
Lansford, Frederick D., Jr., 9
laser therapy, 27
Lavoris, 138, 174, 175, 176, 217
law of expectancy, 158–159
laxatives, 49, 57–62
  for eczema, 242
  lecithin as, 79
  See also internal cleansing
leaky gut syndrome, 2, 5, 6–10
  arthritis and, 236
  "Leaky Gut Syndrome:
    Breaking the Vicious Cycle"
    (Galland), 236
  slippery elm bark tea for,
    115–117
lecithin, 75, 77–80
lemon juice, 75, 94–95

as carbonated beverage
    substitute, 99
in hot water, as coffee substitute, 97
*See also* citrus fruits/juices
Lemon Vinaigrette, 300
Lenoir's Eczema Remedy, 239
lesions
    on face, 178–179
    on hands and feet, 180–193
    during healing process, 194–200,
        215–221
    on scalp, 172–179
    sites of, 21, 26
    thickness of, 19
    *See also* external applications
*Let's Get Well* (Davis), 78
*Let's Live,* 24
lettuce, 108, 224
leukocyte antigen sensitivity test
    (LAST), 103
Lewis, George, 24
Lillard, Harvey, 127
lime juice. *See* lemon juice
"Link a Virus to Arthritis"
    (Randal), 224
Listerine, 137–138, 174, 175, 176
Litt, Jerome Z., 24
liver
    anatomy, 44–45, *45,* 46–47
    carbonated drinks and, 98–99
    hepatic cells, 36
*Living Body, The* (Best, Taylor), 58
"Low-Fat Diet Said to Ease Arthritis"
    (AP), 225
Lucas, Charles P., 225–226
Lugol's Solution, 230
lumen, 7–8
lunch, 279, 283–288
lungs
    anatomy, 42–44, 46–47
    breathing exercises for, 49
lupus erythematosus, 40–41, 233
lymph

high colonic irrigation and, 50
    purifying, 36
maple syrup, 92
Marks, Ronald, 23, 241
Massachusetts General Hospital, 28
massage
    for arthritis, 234, 235
    olive oil–tincture of myrrh for,
        139–140
    Oster whirlpool massager, 183
McGarey, WIlliam A., 228
meal planning
    principles, 277–279
    recipes, 289–302
    sample menus, 283–288
    *See also* diet
Medici family, 148–149
melons, 56, 74, 280
mental formula (Coué), 152–155
methotrexate (MTX), 28, 34–35,
    51, 236
milk, 88–89, 98, 241. *See also* dairy
milk of magnesia, 59
milk thistle, 105
mind. *See* right thinking
minerals
    assimilation of, 74
    supplements, 103–104
molasses, 92
mold, 7
Morfam Master Massager,
    128, 234
mouthwash. *See individual
    product names*
mullein tea, 98, 112, 117–118, 239
"muse" period of self-hypnosis,
    154–155

Nakagawa, S. A., 169
National Academy of Sciences, 61
National Institute on Aging, 170
National Institutes of Health (NIH),
    20, 24, 109

National Psoriasis Foundation (NPF),
    25, 30
natural cathartics. *See* laxatives
negativity
    emotions and, 162–164
    rejecting negative thinking,
        150–152, 264–265
nervous system, 119–120. *See also* spine
neurodermatitis, 161
*New England Journal of Medicine,*
    29–30, 61, 96
*New York Daily News,* 224
*New York Times,* 161–162
nightshades, 7, 68–69
    acid-alkaline balance and, 75
    arthritis and, 226
    dangers of, 80–82
Nightshades Research
    Foundation, 226
No-Nightshade Diet, 226
North American Academy of
    Manipulative Medicine, 126
Norwegian cod liver oil, 236–237
nut allergies, 130, 218
NutraSweet, 93
*Nutritional Influences on Illness*
    (Werbach), 104
nylon clothing, 143

oatmeal bath, 137
Oatmeal-Cinnamon Hotcakes—with
    Variations, 289–290
oils, 83–84
    castor, 45, 59, 114, 132
    cod liver, 236–237
    flaxseed, 108–109
    olive, 45, 53, 60, 83–84, 130–132,
        139–140, 216, 243–244
    omega-3, 108–109, 236–237
    peanut, 130–132, 226–228, 232
    *See also* diet; external applications
ointments. *See* external applications
olive oil

in diet, 83–84
for eczema, 243–244
as laxative, 60
peanut oil mixture with, 45,
    130–132, 216
in Three-Day Apple Diet, 53
in tincture of myrrh massage,
    139–140
omega-3 oils, 108–109, 236–237
omega visualization, 155–156
"1-2-3" concept, 35
oolong tea, 98, 112, 248–249
orange juice "sandwich," 59
Orange Roughy with Spinach,
    Poached, 293
Oriental Chicken Salad, 292–293
O'Rourke, John, 24
osteoarthritis, 223
osteopaths, 123
Oster Hand Massager, 128, 234
Oster whirlpool massager, 183
overeating, 102

Pagano, John O. A., 13
    contact information, 93, 101
    *Dr. John's Healing Psoriasis
        Cookbook . . . Plus!,* 93, 101,
        190, 282
pajama shower/bath, 220–221
Palmer, D. D., 127
palms, 139
paprika, 81, 82
pasta, 91
peaches, 58
Peale, Norman Vincent, 157
peanut allergy, 130, 218
peanut oil, 130–132, 226–228, 232
pears, 58
peppers, 81, 82
perspiratory system, 20–21, 43, 49
    deodorant vs. antiperspirant,
        178–179
    emotions and, 160–161

*Phaedrus* (Plato), 33
phosphatide, 79
phosphoric acid, 78
photochemotherapy, 27, 28
*Physician's Reference Notebook*
    (McGarey), 228
physiotherapy
    electrical stimulation, 138–139,
        234, 235
    techniques to use at home,
        142–143
pizza, 82–83
plastic wrap treatment
    alternative to, 131
    for arthritis, 232
    for hands/feet, 181–182, 183–185,
        190–191
Plato, 33
plicae circulares, 9
Poached Orange Roughy with
    Spinach, 293
Polotchoff, A. G., 161
polyarthritis, 223
pork, 88
portion size, 101, 110, 215
*Positive Imaging* (Peale), 157
Pottenger, Francis M., 36, 47, 50, 77,
    119–120, 168–169
poultry, 86–88
power of thought, 146–147
Prednisone, 7
pregnancy precautions, 113, 116
prescription corticosteroids, 7
prescription hormones, 7
prolapsus of colon, 40
proteins, 276–277
prunes, 58, 73
pruritus. *See* itching
psoralen, 28
psoriasis
    anatomy of digestive tract and,
        4–9, 5, 8
    causes of, 2–3, 4, 10, 26, 125

common types of, 21–23
defined, 2, 17–18
eczema correlation, 246–249
on face, 178–179
future of treatment for,
    267–271
on hands, feet, 180–193
health of patient and, 26–27,
    32–35
incidence of, 24–25
"1-2-3" concept of, 35
recurrence of, 257–261
on scalp, 172–179
T-cells and, 30
treatment success, 1–2, 11–16,
    32–33, 144, 194–195,
    215–221, 254–256
*See also* Cayce/Pagano Regimen;
    diet; external applications;
    healing process; internal
    cleansing; intestinal tract; skin
"Psoriasis and Psoriatic Arthritis
    Treatment Guide, 2004/2005"
    (National Psoriasis
    Foundation), 30
"Psoriasis—Hope for the Afflicted"
    *(ARE Journal)*, 258
Psoriasis Kit (Baar Products), 177
*Psoriasis* (Marks), 23
psoriatic arthritis, 21, 23, 222–223,
    235–236
    acid-alkaline balance and, 72
    Atomodine for, 230
    cyclosporine for, 29–30
    diet and, 224–226, 236–237
    emotions and, 166
    forms of arthritis, 223
    Glyco-Thymoline for, 138, 231
    leaky gut syndrome and, 236
    "poker spine" and, 233–234
    RA-1 virus and, 224
    stress and, 229
    swollen joints from, 231–233

psoriatic arthritis (*continued*)
  treatment regimens for, 226–228,
    234–235
  "winter itch" and, 228–229
  *See also* arthritis
psoriatic spondylitis, 223
*Psychology Today,* 164–165
psyllium husks, 59
purge period, 34–35
purine bodies, 84–86
pustular psoriasis, 21, 22, 187,
    204–205
PUVA (psoralen ultraviolet type A)
    therapy, 28, 51, 268

ragweed allergy, 117
raisins, 58
Randal, Judith, 224
RA-1 virus, 224
Ray's Ointment, 133, 174, 178,
    239, 242
*Reader's Digest,* 104–105
recipes, 289–302. *See also* teas
red meat, 68–69, 88
redundant colon, 37
religious beliefs, 170
repetition, self-hypnosis and, 153
Resinol, 132, 133
restaurants, 106–107
rheumatoid arthritis (RA), 23, 222,
    223, 224, 227
rheumatoid factor, 23
rice
  about, 91–92
  Brown Rice with Lentils,
    294–295
right thinking
  alpha/omega visualization and,
    155–156
  defined, 145–146
  directing thoughts for, 157–158
  imaging and, 156–157
  inner beliefs and, 148–150

law of expectancy and, 158–159
  mental formula of Coué, 152–155
  rejecting negativity and,
    150–152
  thought process and, 147–148
  Troward on power of thought,
    146–147
  *See also* attitude
Roasted Carrots and Parsnips,
    293–294
Roast Turkey Breast, 297
Rockefeller University, 30
romaine lettuce, 108
Rona, Zoltan P., 6–7, 236
rubber gloves, 182–183

saccharin, 93
sacrum, 121–123, *122*
saffron tea. *See* American yellow
    saffron tea
salad dressings, 83–84
salt, 63, 225–226
salves. *See* external applications
sanitation, 47–48
saturated fats, 7
sauna, 135
scalp, 172–179
  hair dryers and, 175
  hair loss and, 173
  overnight oil treatment, 176–178
  psoriasis along hairline, 173–174
  shampoo and electric heat cap
    treatments, 174–176
Schamberg, Jay F., 69
Schweitzer, Albert, 145
scleroderma, 40–41
*Search for God* (Cayce), 171
seeds, 90
self-hypnosis, 153–155
self-image, 169–170
senokot, 58
Sesame Noodles with Kale, 298
shampoo, 172–179

shellfish, 84–86, 185
side dishes, 301–302
sigmoid colon, *37, 38,* 52
Simpson, Robert, 224
sitz bath, 217
skin
  color of, 24
  germinative cell population and,
    19–20
  innervation of, 124
  layers of, 18–19, *19, 20,* 173,
    187–190
  lungs and, 42–44, 46–47
  perspiratory system and, 20–21
slippery elm bark powder, 7–8, 97,
    111–112, 115–117, 239, 264
SMA-12/SMA-24 blood tests, 78
smiling, 171
smoking, 7, 81, 253
snacks, 288
sodium bicarbonate (baking soda)
  as external application, 132, 137
  for laundry, 131–132
Solomon, George F., 161–162
spasm (in colon), *39*
spicy food, 193
spinal adjustment
  manipulation and stimulation,
    *127,* 127–128
  misalignment and, 7
  rationale and technique for,
    125–126
  timing of, 264–265
  *See also* spine; vertebrae
spinal cord, 121, *123*
*Spinal Manipulation* (Bourdillon),
    126
spine, 119–120
  anatomy of, 120–123, *122, 123,*
    *124, 127*
  causes of psoriasis and, 125
  innervation of skin and, 124
  "poker," 233–234

spinal adjustment, 7, 125–128,
    *127,* 223, 239, 264–265
squid, 84
Stanford University, 139
starches, 276–277
steam, teas and, 114, 217
steam baths, 62–63, 135
  for home use, 142
  saffron tea with, 63–64
  witch hazel in, 137–138
steroids, 27
stewed fruits, 58
stomach, *8*
strawberries, 56, 73, 227
stress, 166–167, 229
stretching, 235
stricture (in colon), *39*
subconscious mind, 152–155
subluxations, 120, 121–123, *123*
suggestive therapy, 153–155
Sulflax, 60
sunlight, 135–136
support system, 216, 251
sweat glands. *See* perspiratory
    system
sweet potatoes, 108
sweets, 92–93, 253–254
swimming, 65
swollen joints, 231–233
symmetric oligoarthritis, 223
*Symptoms of Visceral Disease*
    (Pottenger), 36, 77, 119–120
synthetic fabrics, 143, 242–243
systemic (internal) therapy, 27
systemic lupus erythematosus (LE),
    40–41, 233

tar baths, 27
Taylor, Norman, 58
T-cell theory, 30
teas, 97–98, 111–118, 264
  American yellow saffron, 7–8,
    63–64, 97, 111–115, 217, 264

teas (*continued*)
  black, 98
  chamomile, 98, 112, 117
  green, 98, 108
  mullein, 98, 112, 117–118, 239
  oolong, 98, 112, 248–249
  precautions for, 97, 113, 116
  slippery elm bark powder, 7–8, 97,
    111–112, 115–117, 239, 264
  watermelon seed, 98, 112, 118
tests
  blood tests, 78
  for food allergies, 103
  for intestinal permeability
    (leaky gut), 10
  for rheumatoid factor, 233
Thayer's Slippery Elm Lozenges, 115
thought process, 147–148, 265–266.
    *See also* right thinking
Three-Day Apple Diet, 53–56,
    102–103, 263
thyroid, 230
*Tissue Cleansing through Bowel
    Management* (Jensen), 37
tobacco, 81
Tofu and Spinach Soup, 290
tomatoes, 68–69, 81, 183, 185
topical therapy. *See* external
    applications
toxins, 2, 4, 9
  acid-alkaline balance and, 77
  buildup of, 47–49
  detoxification, 49–50, 65–66
  diet and, 107–110
  external applications and, 141–142
  Herxheimer reaction and, 219–221
  negative thoughts as, 265–266
  perspiratory system and, 20–21,
    43, 49, 160–161, 178–179
  toxemia, 47
  *See also* diet; internal cleansing
"Train of Causation" (Troward),
    146–147
transverse colon, *37,* 52

tri-salts, 60, 231
triune approach to health, 34
Tromp, S. W., 80
Troward, Thomas, 146–147, 148, 155
Tufts University, 78, 87

ultrasound, as topical therapy, 138–139
ultraviolet (UV) light therapy, 27, 129
  artificial, 135–136
  lamps for home use, 142
  natural sunlight, 135–136
  types of, 28
undergarments, 143
University of Modena, 61
urea, 41–42
uric acid, 57, 84
urination, 41–42

valves of Kerckring, 9
Vaseline, 132, 133, 174, 178
Vaswani, Dada J. P., 271
vegetables
  above-/below-ground, 275–276
  acid-alkaline balance and, 73–76
  green leafy vegetables, 107
  preparation of, 279
  vegetable juice, 74, 95
  *See also* recipes
vertebrae
  cervical (neck), 121–123, *122, 127*
  dorsal (thoracic), 121–123, *122,
    124, 127, 239*
  intervertebral disks, *122,* 122–123
  lumbar, 121–123, *122, 127,* 239
  middorsal, 120
  vertebral subluxations (vertebral
    lesions), 121–123, *122*
  *See also* spine
vinegar. *See* apple cider vinegar
visualization
  alpha/omega, 155–156
  will and, 148–149
"Vitamin A vs. Psoriasis"
    (O'Rourke), 24

vitamins
    A, 24, 28, 104, 105
    assimilation of, 74
    B, 58, 104
    D, 104
    D, cream, 28–29
    E, 133–134
    supplements, 103–105
    *See also* diet
von Zumbusch's disease, 22

walking, 64–65
water intake, 7, 94–95, 107, 108
    dehydration and, 219–221
    for internal cleansing, 49, 56–57
    kidneys and, 41
    lemon juice and, 75, 94–95, 97, 99
    saffron water, 63, 113
    for "winter itch," 228–229
watermelon seed tea, 98, 112, 118
weather, acid-alkaline balance and,
    80

weight loss, 100–101, 215
Werbach, Melvyn R., 104
wet sauna, 135
whirlpools, 142, 183, 228–229,
    232
white potatoes, 81, 82
white vinegar, 174, 175
whole grains, 61, 89–92, 280
Wilan, Robert, 20
will, imagination and,
    148–150, 155
wine, 99
"winter itch," 228–229
witch hazel, 62, 64, 137–138

yeast, 10
yoga, 43, 235
*Your Skin and How to Live in It*
    (Litt), 24

Zilatone, 59
zinc, 105

# ABOUT THE AUTHOR

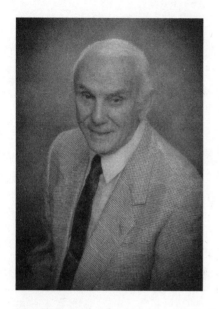

Dr. John O. A. Pagano has been a chiropractic physician in Englewood Cliffs, New Jersey, for forty-eight years. After serving in the navy, he entered the School of Visual Arts in New York City, for medical illustration. His interest shifted to chiropractic. He entered Lincoln Chiropractic College (now National University of Health Sciences) in Lombard, Illinois, graduating with honors in 1959. While interning at a hospital in Denver, Dr. Pagano met his first psoriasis patients. The thought of their torment never left him. He embarked on research that exceeded thirty-five years, proving that psoriasis and eczema can be controlled and healed naturally. The bestseller *Healing Psoriasis: The Natural Alternative* is the culmination of those efforts.

Dr. Pagano has been a featured guest on network television and radio programs such as CNBC's *America's Talking, Jersey's Talking,* NBC's *Unsolved Mysteries, The Ronald Hoffman Show, The Gary Null Show,* WABC's *TALKRadio with Alan Colmes* (of *Hannity & Colmes*), and *Alternative Medicine.* He has lectured throughout the United States, Canada, Asia, Europe, and England, and has appeared before the H.H. Dalai Lama in India. He presented his work at the 2001 World Conference on Psoriasis in San Francisco (National Psoriasis Foundation), the Italian Psoriasis Association in Rome, and the Parapsychology Society of the United Nations.

Dr. Pagano's approach is devoid of drugs (internal or external), tar baths, laser, or ultraviolet light. His regimen focuses on healing the leaky gut syndrome (which he believes causes psoriasis and eczema) through diet, detoxification, and spinal adjustments. The contents of this book are dedicated to that end.